T0143479

The Lived Experience
in Mental Health

The Lived Experience in Mental Health

Gary Morris
Nursing Lecturer, University of Leeds, UK

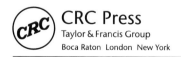

CRC Press
Taylor & Francis Group
Boca Raton London New York

CRC Press is an imprint of the
Taylor & Francis Group, an **informa** business

CRC Press
Taylor & Francis Group
6000 Broken Sound Parkway NW, Suite 300
Boca Raton, FL 33487-2742

© 2017 by Taylor & Francis Group, LLC
CRC Press is an imprint of Taylor & Francis Group, an Informa business

No claim to original U.S. Government works

Printed on acid-free paper
Version Date: 20160603

International Standard Book Number-13: 978-1-4822-4539-4 (Paperback)

This book contains information obtained from authentic and highly regarded sources. While all reasonable efforts have been made to publish reliable data and information, neither the author[s] nor the publisher can accept any legal responsibility or liability for any errors or omissions that may be made. The publishers wish to make clear that any views or opinions expressed in this book by individual editors, authors or contributors are personal to them and do not necessarily reflect the views/opinions of the publishers. The information or guidance contained in this book is intended for use by medical, scientific or health-care professionals and is provided strictly as a supplement to the medical or other professional's own judgement, their knowledge of the patient's medical history, relevant manufacturer's instructions and the appropriate best practice guidelines. Because of the rapid advances in medical science, any information or advice on dosages, procedures or diagnoses should be independently verified. The reader is strongly urged to consult the relevant national drug formulary and the drug companies' and device or material manufacturers' printed instructions, and their websites, before administering or utilizing any of the drugs, devices or materials mentioned in this book. This book does not indicate whether a particular treatment is appropriate or suitable for a particular individual. Ultimately it is the sole responsibility of the medical professional to make his or her own professional judgements, so as to advise and treat patients appropriately. The authors and publishers have also attempted to trace the copyright holders of all material reproduced in this publication and apologize to copyright holders if permission to publish in this form has not been obtained. If any copyright material has not been acknowledged please write and let us know so we may rectify in any future reprint.

Except as permitted under U.S. Copyright Law, no part of this book may be reprinted, reproduced, transmitted, or utilized in any form by any electronic, mechanical, or other means, now known or hereafter invented, including photocopying, microfilming, and recording, or in any information storage or retrieval system, without written permission from the publishers.

For permission to photocopy or use material electronically from this work, please access www.copyright.com (http://www.copyright.com/) or contact the Copyright Clearance Center, Inc. (CCC), 222 Rosewood Drive, Danvers, MA 01923, 978-750-8400. CCC is a not-for-profit organization that provides licenses and registration for a variety of users. For organizations that have been granted a photocopy license by the CCC, a separate system of payment has been arranged.

Trademark Notice: Product or corporate names may be trademarks or registered trademarks, and are used only for identification and explanation without intent to infringe.

Visit the Taylor & Francis Web site at
http://www.taylorandfrancis.com

and the CRC Press Web site at
http://www.crcpress.com

Printed and bound in the United States of America by Publishers Graphics.
LLC on sustainably sourced paper.

To

Herta Kögler – *ein wahrer Held*

and

Emily, Daisy and Caitlin

Lottie, William and Sam

With much love

Contents

Acknowledgements

There are a number of people whom I need to thank without whom I would never have finished (or indeed started) this work.

My wife Emily who has been an invaluable support. Your intuitiveness, insight and creativity have been a major boost to the shaping and structuring of this work.

The many service users and carers who permitted me to access and share their narratives. You are truly 'experts by experience'.

My colleagues Anne Lawton, Julia Turner, Gordon Teal, Shupikai Rinomhota and Nicola Clibbens. Thanks for sharing resources and ideas and allowing me to learn from your experience.

The nursing students who have been involved with this work and engaged with a number of the narratives. You have been fantastic ambassadors showing the difference that lived experience learning can have for practice.

Barry-Percy Smith and Christine Rhodes. Your timely supervision and productive guidance have kept me grounded and focused with regard to the learning strategy featured in this work.

The supportive publishing staff, especially Naomi Wilkinson, Jennifer Blaise, Grace McInness and Vijay Bose. Your help and guidance has been much welcomed.

Thanks to all of you!

List of figures

Introduction

This work is concerned with what it feels like to live with and experience mental health problems. It covers a broad spectrum of experience addressing the internal component of thoughts and emotions. This provides a contextual understanding of a person's daily experiences, encountered difficulties, coping approaches and available support networks. There is a clear need for healthcare professionals and learners to become more aware of and 'tuned in' to the lived and felt experience of those they are engaged with in practice. The importance of this is the promotion of a more caring culture as the more we know about others, the more meaningful and effective our engagement with them becomes. The mental health practitioner's role is built upon core qualities including empathy, genuineness and trust and the ability to develop effective therapeutic relationships. This is built around our ability to appreciate what mental health experience *means* to a person as well as developing an awareness of what it *feels* like. This understanding relates to a person's mental health experience as well as their experience of care. It importantly helps clinicians have better awareness as to why, for example, a person might be struggling to 'comply' with help offered because of problems with medication side effects or anxiety around starting psychological therapies. The contextualisation of this experience allows us to better appreciate difficulties a person is experiencing and 'reframe' from an internal perspective what might otherwise be regarded as 'challenging behaviours'. Acknowledging and appreciating this enables us to respond more appropriately and support people more effectively.

It needs to be noted that the range of mental health lived experience is vast. The work presented here makes no claims about reflecting the totality of this experience or even a small fraction as each person, out of the billions of people affected with mental health issues, will have their own unique narrative to relate. It also needs noting that given the space available in this text and the level of analysis desired, only a select number of mental health issues are featured. These primarily focus upon anxiety, depression, bipolar, psychosis and dementia. Whilst these have been separated out and examined separately within distinct chapters, it needs understanding that in reality there are multiple points of overlap between them. As indicated, this work does not intend to comprehensively understand mental health experience but instead promote thought and encourage a more reflective and questioning approach to practice.

PROCESS

This work is a product of collaborative engagement with service users and carers, those rightfully regarded as 'experts by experience'. The starting point was a series of interviews with individuals about their personal mental health experience. Opinions and experiences were subsequently widened through the distribution of a questionnaire. Initial data were gathered around the experience of mental health problems as well as corresponding care interventions. The focus extended beyond that of experienced difficulties to also encompass recovery and well-being. Generated themes were then further refined and critically reviewed in connection with related research and lived experience resources accessed from a wide selection of media resources. The emergent knowledge and understanding has been fed back and shared with service users in order to verify the authenticity of findings. The result is a textual examination, rich in expressive content illustrating depth and range of experience. A recurring feature within the chapters is the 'personal narrative' boxes which contain examples of direct quotes taken from those interviewed. It can also be noted that the chapter titles are derived from interviewees' comments or personal narratives obtained from media sources.

Permission has kindly been given by many individuals and organisations to share their insightful and thought-provoking narratives to which I am very grateful. A point to clarify is that some of these have been anonymised, with names removed or concealed at the request of those concerned.

STRUCTURE

This work has been divided into three distinct parts. The first part contains two chapters detailing what in essence lived experience narratives entail and the growing involvement of service users in healthcare education. The second part contains the five main chapters focusing directly upon lived mental health experience. Each of these chapters has been split into three distinct sections:

- Section 1: Experience of mental health issue
- Section 2: Experience of care
- Section 3: Well-being

The first section outlines the person's lived and felt mental health experience – essentially what it feels like to, for example, live with depression. This includes difficulties posed through maladaptive attempts to cope, that is, through self-medicating approaches such as drinking or taking drugs. The second part is focused around the person's experience of care with various interventions reviewed such as psychological therapies, medication, in-patient care, creative approaches and peer support. The final section shifts the focus and emphasis from *difficulties* and experiences of *struggling* to that of *coping*. This is concerned with well-being, resilience and recovery, even if a person is still coping with a debilitating condition.

CHAPTER SUMMARY

PART 1: LIVED EXPERIENCE AND LEARNING

CHAPTER 1: EMBRACING LIVED EXPERIENCE

This chapter outlines the importance and need of engaging with the internal world of those living with various mental health problems. It explores the nature of *lived experience* and what this signifies along with the associated term of *narrative*. There is an exploration of the scope of accessible first-person narratives within a variety of media source types and the types of communicative mode employed. A further issue discussed within this chapter considers the validity of personal narratives as 'evidence', linked to the notion of service users being viewed as *experts through experience*.

CHAPTER 2: 'I BECAME INVOLVED TO MAKE A DIFFERENCE': SERVICE USER ENGAGEMENT

The essence of this chapter is an examination of the steadily developing range of service users' involvement in healthcare education. The need can be linked to the promotion of empathic care with clinicians having a greater awareness and understanding around the needs of those they are engaged with in practice. This chapter outlines the historical journey of service user involvement before examining individuals' personal experience of the involvement process.

PART 2: THE LIVED EXPERIENCE IN MENTAL HEALTH

CHAPTER 3: 'STANDING ON A CLIFF EDGE': LIVING WITH ANXIETY

This chapter explores the experience of living with anxiety as related to a range of manifestations including phobias, social anxiety, panic attacks, generalised anxiety, obsessive compulsions and post-traumatic stress. Whilst having a self-protective function, difficulties are experienced where a person's fears become excessive or persistent impacting their ability to cope with daily situations. The experience of living with anxiety is examined along with individuals' responses to various interventions.

CHAPTER 4: 'WALKING IN TREACLE': LIVING WITH DEPRESSION

This chapter is concerned with individuals' experience of lowered mood and a contextualised examination of the term 'depression'. It commences by reflecting upon the point of first recognition of symptoms, seeking help and receiving a diagnosis. Attempts to understand what a person with depression experience entails are made with a critical examination of themes such as numbness, hopelessness, suicidal ideation and isolation.

CHAPTER 5: 'MY BRAIN WON'T SLOW DOWN': LIVING WITH EXTREMES OF MOOD

This builds upon Chapter 4 examining the experience of living with extreme mood states at both ends of the spectrum, including both depressed and elevated. There are however significant differences to the experiences explored in Chapter 4 as having experienced periods of euphoria, high productivity and a sense of heightened awareness, there will be a keen awareness of what is subsequently different or lost when mood significantly lowers. The experience of elevated mood and the disruptive impact this can have upon a person's life will also be explored.

CHAPTER 6: 'THERE'S A STORM INSIDE': LIVING WITH ALTERED REALITY

This chapter is about the experience of *altered reality* and its influence upon a person's life. It is primarily linked here with mental health conditions such as psychosis and schizophrenia. Experiences including delusions and hallucinations are focused upon along with individuals' strategies for coping. Stigma poses particular problems as do co-existing mental health sates of anxiety and depression.

CHAPTER 7: 'PATCHING OVER THE HOLES': LIVING WITH IMPAIRED COGNITION

The themes covered in this chapter reflect the thoughts and feelings involved when coping with an ongoing deterioration in one's capabilities and cognition due to the presence of dementia. It is commonly viewed with negative associations connected with loss of ability, increased confusion and enforced dependency. Available narratives however illustrate a broad range of experience with many examples of people coping and living well with dementia.

PART 3: EMBRACING LIVED EXPERIENCE NARRATIVES

CHAPTER 8: NARRATIVE RESOURCES

This chapter provides examples of some of the many narratives accessible across a broad range of media types. They are grouped according to the mental health conditions covered in Chapters 3 through 7 and complemented with a selection of more generic examples. They are predominantly geared towards the United Kingdom with English language resources although a small range of international products have also been included.

CHAPTER 9: LEARNING STRATEGY

The framework within this chapter provides readers with a strategy of learning concerned with the accessing and processing of lived experience narratives. It is aimed at teaching personnel, workplace trainers and healthcare learners. The strategy outlined here is concerned with a cyclical process of learning engaging successive narrative products. The educational approach covers a strategy for engagement *before*, *during* and *after* the accessing of narrative accounts.

PART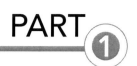

LIVED EXPERIENCE AND LEARNING

Embracing lived experience

INTRODUCTION

This chapter outlines the importance and need of engaging with the internal world of those living with various mental health problems. It reflects upon aspects such as personal narratives, life story work and autobiographical accounts as means of expressing and sharing personal experience. First, the sense of what *lived experience* signifies is reviewed along with the associated term of *narrative*. This is followed by an exploration of the scope of accessible first-person narratives within a variety of media source types. As will be covered, these are conveyed utilising a wide variety of communicative modes such as textual, visual or auditory means. They are very individual expressions and in a number of instances can initially appear confusing or hard to understand. These, however, can be rich in expressive symbolism or visual significance conveying important messages about a person's internal experience, thoughts and feelings. As will be seen throughout this book, the importance of engaging with and connecting with lived experience narratives concerns the opportunity to get closer to and understand more about a person's internal experience. This is vital for carers as effective care can only be delivered if one has understanding as to what a person is feeling or experiencing in relation to various mental health problems. It is also important to have greater awareness as to a person's subjective experience of care interventions. This helps us understand why perhaps a person may not want to continue with their prescribed medication or what their concerns about attending for psychotherapy might be. We can also note what people are telling us that is helpful for them such as the vital feelings of acceptance and connectedness felt through engaging with others who are experiencing mental health problems. A further issue discussed within this chapter considers the validity of personal narratives as 'evidence' which is linked to the notion of service users being *experts through experience*.

WHAT IS LIVED EXPERIENCE?

The concept *lived experience* concerns a person's awareness and comprehension of both internal and external stimuli. This concerns what is occurring inside one or within one's surrounding environment. It involves the capacity to think, feel and perceive what *is* happening and what *has* happened. Wilhelm Dilthey (1985, p. 227) regarded lived experience as having a particular structural nexus and being part of a system of contextually related experiences. These he argued are related to each other like 'motifs in the andante of a symphony'. Our perceptual processing of stimuli can be regarded through Gestalt theory which shows how experience is understood and made sense of (King and Wertheimer, 2007). In this way perceived elements are organised into a unified whole with *closure* or *figure and ground* evaluations being applied. The reading of experience is clearly unique and significant to each person, influenced by both emotive and cognitive processing factors. Past experiences (memories, thoughts and feelings) influence one's subsequent comprehension of what is occurring in the present. What we know or what we feel about specific events or themes has an influence upon how we understand and process them in the present. With regards to mental health issues, there are a number of aspects which will influence a person's subjective experience of what is occurring. Personal or family experience of mental health problems, peer influences, stigmatising attitudes held by others or media reporting will all impact upon one's sense of what one's experience means or signifies. Experiences are unique and personal and can differ significantly from the accounts of others. This applies to what might be regarded as shared experience with narratives around issues such as abuse, trauma or bereavement, or covering a wide spectrum of perspectives. This needs acknowledging when working with service users, and it cannot be assumed even if working extensively with individuals experiencing similar psychological distress that one ever understands the totality of that experience. We can also note here the changing nature of a person's narrative as they progress along a *struggling-coping* continuum. A person with depression, for example, will notice key perceptual differences in how they perceive events as their mood state alters. Expressions of hopelessness and despair can be replaced with a sense of resilience and optimism significantly altering how events are perceived.

NARRATIVE

The term *narrative* is defined by the *Oxford English Dictionary* (2015) as

> A spoken or written account of connected events; a story

This highlights a prominent function involving the chronicling and detailing of experience. Each person will have their own way of detailing what they have encountered. A point of significance concerns *who* it is that is recounting facts and *what* their 'take' or perception of events is, which can give rise to some wildly opposing descriptions. This can be seen in ways in which historical events have been recorded with political or cultural dimensions placing specific evaluations upon what is being expressed. The enduring quality of narrative is expressed by Barthes (1977, p. 79):

> narrative is present in every age, in every place, in every society; it begins with the very history of mankind and there nowhere is, nor has been a people without a narrative ... narrative is international, transhistorical, transcultural; it is simply there, like life itself.

This statement attests to the richness and importance of narrative. It is a fundamental need, something which enables us to signify our existence. This can be reflected against Descartes' (Open University, 2015) Latin proposition *cogito ergo sum* ('I am thinking, therefore I exist'), which signifies that the contemplation of one's existence proves that an 'I' exists to do the thinking. We can reflect this against the situation where one's thinking has become impaired through conditions such as psychosis or dementia. Experience is clearly still being *lived* although the person's concept of what is occurring has become distorted. Whilst we might discount delusional or hallucinatory experience as not being based in reality, the fact that it is not *our* reality does not make it any less real (or distressing) to those experiencing it. A challenge facing healthcare professionals is in finding modes with which to communicate or attend to what is being expressed when content appears confusing or indecipherable. This is where we can consider the variety of communicative types through which narratives can be conveyed, including textual modes, art, music, dance and drama.

Narrative expression concerning what a person is experiencing internally is important in helping carers to better understand and appreciate service users. This provides opportunities to reframe what are rather clumsily referred to as 'challenging behaviours'. Here, internal sensations of feelings act as 'drivers' for a person's externally observed behaviour (O'Connor and Seymour, 1990). Tom Kitwood (1997), relating to dementia care, stressed that there is a reason for all behaviour. This has a strong emotive base with, for example, a person's sense of feeling 'lost' and disconnected contributing towards their agitation and wandering. The issue here concerns a person's ability to correctly comprehend their lived experience and convey it in a comprehensible way. Allied to this is the need for carers to assist individuals with their communication as well as persevering with our attempts to hear what is being conveyed. In some cases this involves developing more creative modes and means of communication as evidenced by John Zeisl's (2009) use of art with people with dementia or the Alzheimer's Society's Singing for the Brain initiative (NHS Choices, 2014). There are narrative and communicative restrictions through many different mental health states with delusional content, memory deficits or dysphasia causing content to appear jumbled and confusing. A person who is depressed may lack the drive to communicate with internal narratives locked firmly inside. We can also consider a person with bipolar with thoughts and speech operating at a speed which others cannot keep up with. As with the examples mentioned earlier, assistance is needed for the person in terms of expressing their narrative as well as for carers to 'hear' what is being said.

In the case of mental health lived experience, other factors besides a person's communicative deficits can restrict their narrative expression. This includes societal attitudes which can feel stigmatising and dismissive as well as a scarcity of opportunities or lack or resources for expression. Enabling the *voice* of those with mental health problems helps to break down barriers and influence acceptance, a crucial need with regard to the levels of discrimination which still prevail. Engaging with personal narratives allows us to begin challenging common stereotypes and misassumptions which proliferate concerning mental health issues, such as the mental health–violence associations or notions around unpredictability and incapability. There is much benefit from asking people how they feel or what they are experiencing as opposed to making assumptions based upon their external behaviour. Mary Shelley's (1818) classic tale *Frankenstein* sums this dynamic up very succinctly as through attending to the creature's narrative we become aware of a sensitive, intelligent being longing for love and affection. He feels cruelly rejected and abandoned by his creator and mocked and abused by those he encounters. Rather than meeting his felt need for compassion he is instead feared, mistrusted and driven away. In a similar vein the responses to people with mental health problems from sections of the media give the impression that what they might be feeling is of far less importance than the emotions of others who feel 'threatened' by their very presence. Poorly informed headlines such as *The Sun's* '1200 Killed by Mental Patients' (Parry and Moyes, 2013) literally scream the notion of *dangerousness* at us. The same newspaper's headlines (Troup, 2003) a few years previously informed us: 'Bonkers Bruno Locked Up'. This grossly insensitive headline totally disregarded the feelings or personal distress experienced to which Frank Bruno (2006, p. 208) later stated:

> I just had no idea how vicious some of the papers could be. I didn't think they'd care so little about the feelings of someone they'd once regarded as a hero ... Now I was a national joke.

Reading Bruno's autobiography, we are given his expressive and detailed account of the occasion when he had required hospital care for his deteriorating mental health state.

NARRATIVES AND COMMUNICATION MODES

There are a number of communicative channels utilised by service users in expressing their lived experience. Some modes are ideally suited for particular emotions or experiences or indeed are personally preferred by different individuals. As Van Manen (1990, p. 71) expresses:

> A poet can sometimes give linguistic expression to some aspect of human experience that cannot be paraphrased without losing a sense of the vivid truthfulness that the lines of the poem are somehow able to communicate. An artist can with a few brushstrokes add depth of emotion to a landscape.

The vibrancy of this statement and the rich variety of communicative modes certainly alert us to the need to be vigilant to what people are communicating and to observe for nuances or levels of expressiveness that may be present even in the most unimagined circumstances. A wonderful example concerns a piece of embroidery filled with narrative text which was completed by a woman with schizophrenia who rarely spoke. The analysis of this item found that although she was silent, she was connected in many ways to the environment around her (Blakeman and Samuelson, 2013). This bears testament to the many unique ways in which narratives can be expressed which also includes modes such as textual (autobiographical reflection, poetry and fiction), visual (painting, drawing and sculpture), auditory (music and song) and performance (dance and theatre). This is evidently not a definitive list as other approaches will be used by individuals given their preference or maybe defined by the restrictions placed upon them by external circumstances or perhaps disability or infirmity. As seen with the embroidered narrative there can be rich forms of expression locked within a person simply requiring an outlet. This can be related to the example of Christy Brown (1954), severely disabled through cerebral palsy and only able to communicate through typing with his *left foot*. When given the opportunity to communicate what emerged was an intelligent, articulate and highly expressive person. The message here was clearly to keep searching for ways and means of facilitating expression.

Each narrative mode has its own special points of emphasis be they vocal cues, facial expressions, brush strokes, harmonisation or symbolism. All of these place special emphasis and stress upon what is being expressed and taken collectively can provide vivid and detailed accounts of a person's lived experience. This is where others are able to get closer to what it feels like to perhaps

- Feel totally numbed and unable to feel pleasure even when, for example, experiencing great success
- Be given a diagnosis of dementia
- Feel threatened and tormented by unseen predators whom only you are aware of
- Be avoided by others who are mistrustful of you

When considering different narrative styles, we can also reflect upon our ability to embrace communication which alters significantly from conventional forms of expression. We might consider here the *language of madness*, a term applied to Jonathan Swift's (1704) *A Tale of a Tub*, which eventually reveals the narrator as a 'madman'. Similarly, Doris Lessing's (1971) *Briefing for a Descent into Hell* and perhaps Bernlef's (1988) *Out of Mind* provide striking first-person accounts expressing the distorted thinking of someone who has been adversely affected by their mental health state. Rich symbolism, abstract imagery and imaginative discourse can make narratives uniquely personal and highly impactful.

ACCESSING NARRATIVES

We can access narratives around mental health lived experience from a variety of sources. A primary source involves practice experience where narratives are relayed first-hand by those experiencing mental health difficulties or from others such as relatives, carers or healthcare professionals. Second-hand accounts are less reliable on account of facts and details which become lost or distorted through being retold, as each person's interpretation is brought to bear. Another rich source or lived experience narratives concern the media with its vast array of documented examples. This includes television documentary, Internet blogs and discussion forums, newspaper or magazine features, films, autobiographies, works of art, along with many others. The communicative mode or form of expression may determine what is prominently conveyed and can also set the tense with which narratives are expressed, for example, present or past. There can be some very strong experiences of, for example, watching a film and having a narrative experience portrayed in the *here and now*. This enables us to experience events and feelings along with narrators, identifying strongly with them and better contextualising the totality of their experience.

WHY DO WE NEED LIVED EXPERIENCE NARRATIVES?

Embracing and understanding more about lived mental health experience facilitates the development of effective partnership work with service users and carers. The importance of this can be reflected against the Francis inquiry report findings (The Mid Staffordshire NHS Foundation Trust Inquiry, 2013) which identified widespread institutional deficiencies and a poor care culture being demonstrated in the services examined. This has implications for all care environments with recommendations being made for an increased patient-centred focus. We can also consider the DoH's (2012) *Compassion in Practice* which advocated an enhanced approach to what is meant by *caring*. The importance of recognising the needs of service users and engaging them more proactively within the care process is a core feature as advocated by notable theorists and researchers such as Carl Rogers (1951), Tom Kitwood (1997) and Hildegard Peplau (1988) whose work has substantially influenced current approaches to mental healthcare. A central proposition advocates the service user being central to the care process with attention given to their subjective experience, day-to-day encounters, thoughts and feelings. The need to get closer to, engage with and better appreciate service users' lived experience is a key component of the mental healthcare practitioner's approach. It reflects the process of empathy which can be regarded as

> the single most important human and technical tool at the therapist's disposal
>
> Strupp (1996, p. 137)

This was also placed centrally by Rogers (1986) as one of the core conditions leading towards healing. The value and significance of life stories/personal narratives for learning about mental health experience is signified by Van Manen (1990, p. 70):

- Provides us with possible human experiences
- Enables us to experience life situations, feelings, emotions, and events that we would not normally experience
- Allows us to broaden the horizons of our normal existential landscape by creating possible worlds
- Tends to appeal to us and involve us in a personal way
- Is an artistic device that lets us turn back to life as lived, whether fictional or real
- Evokes the quality of vividness in detailing unique and particular aspects of a life that could be my life or your life
- Transforms lived experience into poetic or symbolic language

These elements show many reasons for healthcarers to embrace and attend to service users' lived experience.

EXPERTS BY EXPERIENCE

An issue which perhaps needs addressing concerns the validity of service user narratives as forms of evidence around mental health experience. The first thing to mention is that each account is unique to the person expressing it and documents what they as individuals are going through and their associated thoughts and feelings. This cannot be known with any certainty by external observers. Historically, the views of service users tended to be overlooked in favour of experienced and trained professionals or researchers. This placed the notion of *expertise* upon others whose knowledge and wisdom was deferred to. This is now changing with recognition being given to the concept of *experts by experience* which credits knowledge acquired through the experience of distress or through caring for someone with mental health problems (CQC, 2013; DoH, 2001). The expression about what this *distress* means relates to the unique insights that personal experience provides. It is the service user who can more accurately convey and contextualise what it feels like to live with certain mental health states. As Evans (1999, p. 9) states this expertise is

> gained not from colleges and formal learning, but from the 24 hour day, day in, day out, experiences of needing to use services for personal support.

Terry (2013) reviewed the partnership work between service users and healthcare educators and concluded that service users and carers are an under-utilised resource and, as experts by experience, have much to offer students and staff by increased involvement in nurse education programmes. These 'experts' can teach us much about what it feels like to perceive oneself as having mental health problems and how day-to-day life and relationships are impacted upon. There are a number of initiatives capitalising upon this experience and providing opportunities for sharing lived experience accounts. A notable resource is provided by the Healthtalk online programme which provides narrated interviews in video, audio and transcript form (Herxheimer and Ziebland, 2004). There are also a number of regional projects including the *Changing Minds* mental health awareness training programme in South London with service users operating as co-trainers (McKinley and Yiannoullou, 2012). Age UK's (2015) *Acting Together* involves *experts by experience* who provide support and information about the experience of living with or caring for someone with dementia. Time to Change appoints 'champions', 'experts through experience' and celebrity ambassadors as well as running an innovative human library initiative. This is also provided by a number of local Trusts, providing the public with individuals who can be consulted about lived mental health experience and their associated thoughts and feelings.

SERVICE-USER LIVED EXPERIENCE

There have been a number of studies examining the lived experience of individuals with mental health problems. These include the experience of being cared for: in forensic psychiatric wards (Horberg et al., 2012), with community treatment orders (Light et al., 2014), through the development and use of a relapse prevention with individuals with bipolar (Daggenvoorde et al., 2013), and in dual diagnosis (bipolar disorder and substance use) (Ward, 2011). Other accounts detail the experience of being treated with psychoactive drugs by women with schizophrenia (Song, 2011) and the meaning of illness to those diagnosed with early-stage dementia (Harman and Clare, 2006). From a mental health perspective, lived experience concerns a variety of factors. First, the contextual understanding and awareness as to what it means to live with, for example, bipolar disorder, depression or dementia. This is a fluid and changing dynamic as personal narratives attest to with a multitude of different examples available. These express vast-ranging experience across a spectrum from positions of vulnerability, despair and helplessness through to those of resilience, strength and coping. We can compare, for example, descriptive terms such as *person suffering with psychosis* with *person living well with psychosis*. This takes us into a person's subjective experience and can challenge personal expectations or stereotypical notions. As will be seen throughout this book, engaging with lived experience means acknowledging mental health issues from a balanced viewpoint examining what distress means as well as appreciating a developing sense of resilience. As Hanson and Mitchell (2001) state, attending to narratives where people are coping can show the degrees of recovery that are possible and aid in dispelling some of the negative associations relating to people with mental health problems. The championing of mental health lived experience is promoted by many service-user advocacy groups, recognising the educative and health promotional benefits. A prime initiative concerns the Time to Change anti-stigma campaign which is run by two major mental health charities, Rethink Mental Illness and Mind. They have a range of champions, people with *lived experience of mental health problems* who are involved in challenging attitudes and behaviours through sharing their own personal experience. One particularly important resource concerns peer support opportunities for sharing experience and promoting understanding such as the discussion forums provided by various mental health advocacy groups including Alzheimer's Society, Bipolar UK, Hearing Voices Network, OCD Action and Mind. A key issue here relates to shared understanding, the sense of being more tuned in to others by nature of shared experience. Gilbert and Stickley's (2012) study of 'wounded healers' highlighted how personal mental health experience can aid understanding of others who are going through a related similar experience. There was a strong sense that study participants believed that their own experiences are instrumental in informing their practice and assisting with empathic responses. Indeed, peer support in mental healthcare and learning is being increasingly recognised and valued (Bassett et al., 2010). This includes a service-user-led advocacy group working with people experiencing complex mental health needs: the Scottish Government's (2009) commissioning of peer support workers and the Cambridgeshire and Peterborough NHS Foundation Trusts (2014).

REFERENCES

Age UK (2015). Acting Together. http://www.ageuk.org.uk, accessed 21 November, 2015.

Alzheimer's Society. (2015). TalkingPoint Forum. http://www.alzheimers.org.uk, accessed 12 September, 2015.

Barthes, R. (1977). Introduction to the structural analysis of narratives. In R. Barthes (Ed.), *Image-Music-Text* (pp. 79–124). Collins: Glasgow, Scotland.

Bassett, T., Faulkner, A., Repper, J. and Stamou, E. (2010). Lived experience leading the way: Peer support in mental health. Together for mental health. http://www.together-uk.org, accessed 18 September, 2015.

Bernlef, J. (1988). *Out of Mind*. Faber & Faber: London, UK.

Bipolar UK. (2015). e-community. http://www.bipolaruk.org.uk, accessed 12 September, 2015.

Blakeman, J.R. and Samuelson, S.J. (2013). Analysis of a silent voice: A qualitative inquiry of embroidery created by a patient with schizophrenia. *Journal of Psychosocial Nursing and Mental Health Services*. 51(6), 38–45.

Brown, C. (1954). *My Left Foot*. Vintage: London, UK.

Bruno, F. (2006). *Bruno: Fighting Back*. Yellow Jersey Press: London, UK.

Cambridgeshire and Peterborough NHS Foundation Trust (2014). Peer support workers. http://www.cpft.nhs.uk/, accessed 5 October, 2015.

Care Quality Commission (2013). Experts by experience programme. http://www.cqc.org.uk/, accessed 6 December, 2014.

Daggenvoorde, T.H., Goossens, P.J. and Gamel, C.J. (2013). Regained control: A phenomenological study of the use of a relapse prevention plan by patients with a bipolar disorder. *Perspectives in Psychiatric Care.* 49(4), 235–242.

Department of Health [DoH] (2001). Mental Health National Service Framework (and the NHS Plan) Workforce Planning, Education and Training Underpinning Programme: Adult Mental Health Services: Final Report by the Workforce Action Team. Department of Health: London, UK.

Department of Health [DoH] (2012). Compassion in practice. http://www.england.nhs.uk.

Dilthey, W. (1985). *Poetry and Experience. Selected Works.* Princeton University Press: Princeton, NJ.

Evans, C. (1999). Gaining our voice: The developing pattern of good practice in user involvement. *Managing Community Care.* 7(2), 7–13.

Gilbert, P. and Stickley, T. (2012). "Wounded healers": The role of lived experience in mental health education and practice. *The Journal of Mental Health Training, Education and Practice.* 7(1), 33–41.

Hanson, B. and Mitchell, D. (2001). Involving mental health service users in the classroom: A course of preparation. *Nurse Education in Practice.* 1(2), 120–126.

Harman, G. and Clare, L. (2006). Illness representations and lived experience in early stage dementia. *Qualitative Health Research.* 16(4), 484–502.

Hearing Voices Network. (2015). Forum. http://www.hearing-voices.org, accessed 12 September, 2015.

Herxheimer, A. and Ziebland, S. (2004). The DIPEx project: Collecting personal experiences in illness and healthcare. In B. Hurwitz, T. Greenhaigh and V. Skultans (Eds.), *Narrative Research in Health and Illness* (pp. 115–131). Blackwell Publishing: Oxford, UK.

Horberg, U., Sjogren, R. and Dahlberg, K. (2012). To be strategically struggling against resignation: The lived experience of being cared for in forensic psychiatric care. *Issues in Mental Health Nursing.* 33(11), 743–751.

King, D.B. and Wertheimer, M. (2007). *Max Wertheimer and Gestalt Theory.* Transaction Publishers: New Brunswick, NJ.

Kitwood, T. (1997). *Dementia Reconsidered.* Open University Press: Buckingham, UK.

Lessing, D. (1971). *Briefing for a Descent into Hell.* Panther: St Albans, England.

Light, E.M., Robertson, M.D., Boyce, P., Carney, T., Rosen, A., Cleary, M. et al. (2014). The lived experience of involuntary community treatment: A qualitative study of mental health consumers and carers. *Australasian Psychiatry.* 22(4), 345–351.

McKinley, S. and Yiannoullou, S. (2012). Changing minds: Unleashing the power of mental health. In M. Barnes and P. Cotterell (Eds.), *Critical Perspectives on User Involvement* (pp. 115–128). The Policy Press: Bristol, UK.

Mind. (2015). elefriends. http://www. mind.org.uk, accessed 12 September, 2015.

NHS Choices (2014). Dementia: Singing for the brain. http://www.nhs.uk, accessed 16 April, 2015.

OCD Action. (2015). Forum. http://www.ocdaction.org.uk/, accessed 12 September, 2015.

O'Connor, J. and Seymour, J. (1990). *Introducing Neuro-Linguistic Programming – Psychological Skills for Understanding and Influencing People.* Aquarian: London, UK.

Open University (2015). Rene Descartes – "I think, therefore I am". http://www.open.edu, accessed 8 November, 2015.

Oxford English Dictionary (2015). Narrative. http://www.oed.com/, accessed 20 March, 2016.

Parry, R. and Moyes, S. (7 October 2013). 1200 killed by mental patients. *The Sun.* Retrieved from http://www.thesun.co.uk, accessed 15 October, 2015.

Peplau, H. (1988). *Interpersonal Relations in Nursing.* Springer Publishing Company: New York.

Rethink Mental Illness. (2015). Time to change. http://www.rethink.org/, accessed 18 September, 2015.

Rogers, C. (1951). *Client-Centered Therapy: Its Current Practice, Implications and Theory.* Constable: London, UK.

Rogers, C. (1986). A client-centered/person-centered approach to therapy. In I. Kutash and A. Wolf (Eds.), *Psychotherapist's Casebook* (pp. 197–208). Jossey-Bass: San Francisco, CA.

Scottish Government Social Research (2009). Evaluation of the delivering for mental health peer support worker pilot scheme. http://www.gov.scot/, accessed 12 August, 2014.

Shelley, M. (1818). *Frankenstein.* Penguin: London, UK.

Song, E.J. (2011). The lived experience of the women with schizophrenia taking antipsychotic medication. *Journal of Korean Academy of Nursing.* 41(3), 382–392.

Strupp, H.H. (1996). Some salient lessons from research and practice. *Psychotherapy.* 33(1), 135–138.

Swift, J. (1704). *A Tale of a Tub.* George Routledge & Sons: London, UK.

Terry, J.M. (2013). The pursuit of excellence and innovation in service user involvement in nurse education programmes: Report from a travel scholarship. *Nurse Education in Practice.* 13(3), 202–206.

The Mid Staffordshire NHS Foundation Trust Public Inquiry (2013). Report of the Mid Staffordshire NHS Foundation Trust Public Inquiry: Executive summary. Stationery Office: London, UK.

Time to Change. (2015). Time to change. http://www.time-to-change.org.uk, accessed 18 September, 2015.

Troup, J. (23 September 2003). Bonkers Bruno locked up. *The Sun* (pp. 1–7). Retrieved from http://www.thesun.co.uk.

Van Manen, M. (1990). *SUNY Series, The Philosophy of Education: Researching Lived Experience: Human Science for an Action Sensitive Pedagogy.* State University of New York Press: New York.

Ward, T.D. (2011). The lived experience of adults with bipolar disorder and comorbid substance use disorder. *Issues in Mental Health Nursing.* 32(1), 20–27.

Zeisl, J. (2009). *I'm Still Here.* Penguin: London, UK.

'I became involved to try to make a difference'
Service user engagement

INTRODUCTION

It is important for learners and healthcare practitioners to develop an awareness and understanding of the lived experiences of those they are engaged with in practice. This helps promote empathic, sensitive and caring approaches to care as strongly advocated by a number of key sources including the Francis Inquiry Report (The Mid Staffordshire NHS Foundation Trust Inquiry, 2013), the 5-Year Mental Health plan (DoH, 2014) and the National Dementia Strategy (DoH, 2009). Learning about lived experience and accessing narrative accounts can be facilitated through various means involving service user engagement in practice and educational environments or exposure to selected media products. This provides opportunities to 'tune in' to personal accounts of living with varied mental health states. The first part of this chapter looks at the historical journey tracing the emergence of the service user as a key factor within healthcare education. The second part is concerned with the personal experience of one's involvement with learning. This is based around a series of interviews and questionnaires by the author which elicited personal reflections around one's involvement. Selected narrative responses representing individuals' views are italicised and included after each question. This is complemented by a review of the effectiveness of this involvement from a learning point of view with related literature accessed.

HISTORICAL DEVELOPMENT

There has been a steady development in emphasis upon service user involvement in practice and education since the early 1990s. *The NHS and Community Care Act* (DoH, 1990) was the first piece of UK legislation to establish a formal requirement for user involvement in service planning. Subsequent key policies in the early 1990s include *The Patient's Charter* (DoH, 1991); *Local Voices* (NHS Management Executive, 1992); *Working in Partnership* (DoH, 1994); *Building Bridges* (DoH, 1995); *The Expert Patient: A New Approach to Chronic Disease Management for the 21st Century* (DoH, 2001a) and the *NHS Improvement Plan* (DoH, 2004). Within this period, 'patient and public involvement' in healthcare became one of the central tenets of New Labour's NHS modernisation agenda (Kemp, 2010), which was formalised in policy terms through the *NHS Plan* emphasising the government's commitment to creating a patient-centred NHS with service users' needs central to service design and delivery (DoH, 2000). Further work has been done

---

Level 5 – Partnership

Service users and teaching staff work collaboratively across a variety of strategic and operational areas. Service users have secure contracts.

Level 4 – Collaboration

Service users as full-time department members are involved in *three* major aspects of faculty work. The department has a statement of values and training/supervision is offered.

Level 3 – Growing involvement

Service users are involved in *two* of the following: planning, teaching delivery, student selection, assessment, management or evaluation. Payment is provided at normal visiting lecturer rates. Training and support offered.

Level 2 – Limited involvement

Service users invited in to 'tell their stories' in a designated slot. No opportunity to shape the course involved. Payment offered.

Level 1 – No involvement

Curriculum planned, delivered and managed with no service user involvement.

Figure 2.1 Ladder of involvement. (From Tew, J. et al., *A Good Practice Guide. Learning from Experience,* Involving service users and carers in mental health education and training, Mental Health in Higher Education, NIMH, Nottingham, UK, 2004.)

with *Transforming Participation in Health and Care* (NHS England, 2013). Within mental healthcare, service user involvement has been promoted through legislative and practice initiatives such as the *National Service Framework for Mental Health* (DoH, 1999) and the *Mental Capacity Act* (DoH, 2005). Professional recognition of the value that service users' experience has for healthcare education can be seen in the NMC's (2010) *Standards for Pre-Registration Nurse Education* which advocates the involvement of service users and carers in the planning, delivery, teaching and evaluation of nursing curricula. The NMC's (2010) standards for pre-registration nurse education in the United Kingdom promote the involvement of service users and carers in the planning, delivery, teaching and evaluation of nursing curricula. This is complemented by recommendations for practitioners to work with service users through a partnership approach (NICE, 2011; NMC, 2015). Such initiatives reflect the developing service user's journey from passive care recipient to active teaching role (McKeown et al., 2010), a progression illustrated by Tew et al.'s (2004) 'ladder of involvement' (see Figure 2.1).

PEER-LED INITIATIVES

The developments addressed here reflect recognition of the expertise and educative value that service users can offer. The enhanced emphasis upon service user involvement through legislative and practice initiatives is matched by the growing status and influence from service user organisations. The number of groups and bodies are steadily increasing as is their influence and impact. Organisations such as Mind, Rethink Mental Illness, the

Alzheimer's Society and the Samaritans are notable examples which are frequently featured within news reports providing expert opinion. Indeed, their responses to high profile media stories help to look more objectively and sensitively at issues affecting people with mental health problems. The furore caused over Tesco and Asda's grossly insensitive 'mental health' Halloween costumes and discriminatory reporting of the German Wings air disaster are two such examples where stigmatising and stereotypical content was publicly challenged by mental health advocacy groups.

SERVICE USER INVOLVEMENT

This part details the experience of service users and carers concerning their involvement within healthcare education. Each question is followed by a box containing italicised text providing examples of responses from service users and carers interviewed. The sentiments expressed are subsequently examined along with related research studies and associated literature.

WHAT HAS YOUR INVOLVEMENT IN HEALTHCARE EDUCATION INCLUDED?

> **Interview narratives**
>
> *A wide range of elements listed which relate to student selection, interviewing, teaching, simulated patient work, assessment, course planning and evaluation, curriculum design, programme validation, practice development, research and conference presentations.*
>
> *'I feel that my past experience, in terms of professional qualifications, experience in industry, technical education, local government, environmental control, and industrial consultancy is hardly used. Perhaps you could have a good database of our skills, so that you can call on us by agreement when a role crops up.'*

The responses here highlight an extensive breadth of involvement with many of these elements broken down into a further range of specific examples. For example, *teaching* has been offered through approaches which include video work, lecturing, role play, online learning packages and group discussion. A key observation regarding the range and scope of involvement is that it extends far beyond the confines of the classroom setting with student engagement and knowledge dissemination occurring in many arenas. The increased participation by service users is illustrated by Weinstein (2010) concerning all aspects of health and social care delivery, planning and professional training. It is notable that the educative role covers the whole span of a students' learning from initial recruitment and selection through to the point of registration. This is heartening to note and validates policy support for greater involvement of both mental health service users and carers throughout the whole education and training process (DoH, 2001b). The partnership work with educational staff is shown through aspects such as curriculum design and programme evaluation with a valuable body of expertise being brought to bear. There are concerns however regarding the large number of courses which are planned and delivered without consultation or input from service users (Higgins et al., 2011). Nickeas (2007), who works as a service user trainer, questions why the overall scale of involvement is so inconsistent and variable in quality feeling that whilst service users have to take responsibility the main emphasis rests with the professionals. This is where the positive promotional work which is being done needs to extend along with recognition of its value.

The expertise held by service users extends into many areas. As found through the interview and questionnaire responses many individuals had professional and technical skills alongside their learning from personal health experiences. Some had worked as teachers, managers or researchers or had extensive experience of health and illness through years of caring for family members. Accordingly, contributions for teaching and learning, course design, practice development and research can be of very high value. From a research perspective, benefits of involving service users include the valuable perspective that can be brought, shaped by people's own experiences (Spiers et al., 2005).

WHAT WAS YOUR REASON FOR YOU GETTING INVOLVED?

Interview narratives

Previous personal experience of poor care – I wanted to educate upcoming practitioners how to understand and improve their service.

I became involved to make services better and try to make a difference.

The realization that some sort of 'work related activity' was good for my psychological and social health.

Retired and want to put my skills to use in the community.

Responses to this question demonstrated a high degree of motivation and commitment to get involved, particularly concerning the opportunity to influence mental healthcare learning and practice. It demonstrated the belief that individuals had something of value to offer as well as perceiving tangible benefits for themselves. This reflects findings by Minogue and Handy (2010) where service users and carers highlighted their reasons for getting involved as wishing to give something back, improve services as well as gain knowledge and develop new skills. There are a number of elements of note here with clear gains and benefits for different parties involved. This sense of 'trade-off' is important and highlights some important implications for those concerned. First, the issue regarding what service users have to offer concerns the already noted *experts by experience* and the opportunity for learners to access a vital and clearly needed perspective. Recognition of this can validate and acknowledge the worth of what a person has to offer, a key factor linked with recovery and developing resilience. This can be reflected against the wide range of awareness raising and supportive initiatives that service users are getting involved with. Discussion Forums such as the Alzheimer's Society's Talking Point Forum or Bipolar UK's e-community show many instances of individuals offering help and advice based upon their own mental health experiences. Here, service users are engaged with others through different positions of *vulnerability* and *resilience*, asking for help and advice as well as giving it. There are many comments attesting to the value of this help. For those giving it, there can be a renewed sense of purpose, productivity and feeling needed, which are central to an individual's sense of well-being. This reflects the Mental Health Foundation's (2003) view that service user involvement can be therapeutic, helping to increase confidence, raise self-esteem and develop new skills. Minogue et al. (2005) showed the benefits for service users as including the gaining of knowledge and experience as well as an improved sense of well-being, self-esteem and confidence. This can be related to the knowledge and recognition that one can make a difference and have the capacity and experience with which to influence practice. It is interestingly to note that the desire to improve care for future generations appears to be influenced through both good and bad personal experiences. Whichever the case may be, both of these experience types have much to offer and teach future healthcare professionals.

To what degree do you feel your expertise has been valued?

Interview narratives

It varies from professional to professional. Sometimes I feel I am tolerated rather than listened to.

I feel 100% valued.

At times it feels like you are taken out of your box for a session and then put back in it.

We get excellent feedback from the students who find it very valuable in their learning.

You can tell your story – whether they take notice who knows.

We know our input is valued because of the increasing work we are being involved in.

Whilst the majority of responses indicated that service users had felt valued there were some notable examples whereby individuals felt uncertain or disappointed about the responses given. A central element here concerns feedback, a vital mechanism for gauging recipients' views and feelings about one's input. Where feedback has been received this has mainly been favourable which is heartening and motivating as well as enabling service users to develop and modify subsequent input. The educational value of service user input for both students and academics is borne out by the available literature. This relates to student nurse selection and recruitment (Rhodes and Nyawata, 2011) and student learning (Khoo et al., 2004; O'Donnell and Gormley, 2013; Schneebeli et al., 2010). The importance of involvement is also acknowledged by service users (Beresford, 2015; Crepaz-Keay, 2012; Morgan and Jones, 2009). The practice need is illustrated through the enhanced empathy towards people with mental health difficulties (Bassman, 2000; Perry et al., 2013) as well as attitudes being challenged and better understanding developed (Minogue et al., 2009; Simons et al., 2007). As Perry et al. (2013) found, it can also break down barriers of stigma with improved attitudes towards people with mental health difficulties. This reflects McAndrew and Samociuk's (2003) findings that involve service users in training that have the potential to challenge some of the myths surrounding mental illness and to enable those responsible for delivering mental health services to gain an insight into what it is like to be on the receiving end of such services. A study by Rush (2008) outlined five mechanisms that contributed to the students' learning which included hearing lived experience narratives, the emotional impact, the reversal of roles, opportunities for reflection and the training/preparation for service users. Notably, learning from service users in the classroom was found to be qualitatively different from learning in clinical placements.

It is clear from the available evidence base that service users have much of value to offer from an educational perspective. It is worrying therefore to note comments about engagement feeling as if it is part of a 'tick box' exercise. This is where involvement is felt to be carried out more for show purposes than for any real educational value. In some instances this process might well feel dissatisfying for all parties involved where educational staff have not effectively planned input with service users or considered the relevance to learners' needs at the stage they are at in their learning. This, as McKeown et al. (2010) point out, is where input can be regarded as tokenistic. This is borne out by a number of studies whereby participants have not felt as if their contributions were valued by teaching staff (Clarke and Holttum, 2013; Meehan and Glover, 2007). An aspect to consider though is the importance of feedback. It might be the case in a number of instances that service users feel uncertain about the value of their input which is actually highly regarded by students but without the mechanisms to feed this back. Educators therefore need to be more mindful of the whole process and remain sensitive to the needs of those getting involved, engaging them more proactively in the whole process from planning through to session evaluation.

WHAT DIFFICULTIES HAVE YOU EXPERIENCED WITH YOUR INVOLVEMENT?

Interview narratives

I have been a member for many, many years without any contact at all. Recently, I have had some involvement but felt I have had to shout about it.

Difficult finding out about how to get involved and who to contact.

Getting paid – very bureaucratical.

All depends on how I feel on the day.

Whilst the majority of respondents stated that they had not encountered any significant difficulty there were some recurrent themes for others. First, we can consider the difficulty of 'breaking in' and feeling part of an already established organisation and staff group. Speed et al.'s (2012) study into potential barriers to becoming engaged in nurse education identified six themes: not knowing the context of the group, lack of preparation of the group, not being supported, not being allowed to be real, not receiving feedback and not being paid appropriately. Some comments illustrated levels of frustration around times of low involvement. A core issue to bear in mind here is that these responses are from individuals already involved within education in higher education and there will no doubt be many who are not able to make any contacts. A large number of respondents were approached by educational staff with input requested. Basset et al. (2006) outline 10 barriers to the involvement of service users in learning and teaching about mental health in higher education along with suggestions for overcoming them (see Figure 2.2).

As Minogue and Handy (2010) found, a number of service users find it hard to get involved preferring a personal approach to that of proactively seeking opportunities themselves or responding to adverts. This can be matched by an obstacle raised by Basset et al. (2006) in that many academics do not know how to access service users and carers. A consequence of this is a select few individuals becoming over-used, thereby limiting the

---

- **Hierarchies that exclude**
Resistance to the involvement of service user involvement with perceived dangers amongst educationalists in letting go a little of the 'expert role'.

- **Stigma and discrimination**
Service users may be regarded as 'ill' all the time or regarded as an exotic being brought into the classroom for students to observe.

- **Validation and accreditation processes**
Service users can feel disempowered and confused by acronyms and jargon. Can be experienced as bullying.

- **Academic jargon and 'put downs'**
It is acknowledged that academic 'put downs' can make a person feel stupid.

- **Clever people/clever excuses**
Endless deliberation, never-ending consultation with well-argued excuses based upon 'evidence'.

- **Knowledge as king and topics/levels**
A lot of higher education teaching is related to theoretical learning and not understanding of personal experience.

- **Individual and not team approach**
There may be few initiatives which cross boundaries between the training of different mental health professionals.

- **Gaining access in the first place**
Educationalists may not know who to approach or who might want to be involved. Equally service users may not know whom to contact.

- **Bureaucratic payment systems**
Involves barriers and delays experienced with payment. Organisations can have inflexible payment systems.

- **Lack of support for trainers/educators**
Service users can feel vulnerable in teaching roles. It can be anxiety-provoking facing a room full of students.

Figure 2.2 Barriers to the involvement of service users.

range of voices which can be heard and potentially feeling unrepresentative. As El Enany et al. (2013) found, those selected tended to be more articulate and able to work with professionals causing concerns about the 'representativeness' of individual service users who may appear 'too well', 'too articulate' or 'too vocal' to be generalisable. This was also voiced by students in Perry et al.'s (2013) study concerning particular service users teaching them. Lindow (1999, p. 166) however suggests that the concept of 'representativeness' may be utilised as a subconscious method of resisting user involvement:

> We ask, would workers send their least articulate colleague to represent their views, or the least confident nurse to negotiate for a change in conditions?

Problems raised by respondents include negotiating bureaucratic hurdles and actually getting paid. Difficulties relate to a lack of clarity around the regulations concerning payment and the set amount that can be earned without benefits being affected (McPhail, 2008; Turner and Beresford, 2005). Another pertinent issue concerns how individuals might be feeling. Participants in De Coster et al.'s (2011) study limited their involvement concerning what they felt able to be involved with given the stage of their recovery process. This raises points of sensitivity concerning what we are asking others to do and an awareness of how well they are feeling. We are after all expecting people in some instances to reveal very personal, intimate and potentially distressing details about themselves.

To what degree would you say your involvement has been a true partnership?

Interview narratives

It is a true partnership because my skills are appreciated and used. I am treated with respect and dignity. I feel valued and because of this I feel confident to speak to students and staff.

I have felt very involved, valued and of equal importance. My views have been taken seriously and my input has been influential.

I think there are some clinician teachers who do not fully appreciate the value of real patients/carers working in medical education.

Sometimes feel when sitting on the interview panel that we are not always given the credit we deserve.

Respondents strongly indicated feeling valued and respected and to a large degree treated as an equal. However, this did not apply to all with some having the experience of feeling of lesser value. As Tait and Lester (2005) highlight, organisations which encourage involvement show commitment to genuine partnerships between service users and healthcare professionals. Such settings generally achieve a more equitable balance of power between service users and staff. As shown by Hitchen et al. (2011), significant difficulties with involvement relate to overcoming professional language barriers and the power imbalances felt between themselves and professionals. This might be due to the problems encountered by some professionals who find it difficult to view service users as 'experts' and resist moves towards greater service user involvement. Although there is evidence to suggest that professionals are generally supportive of user involvement, there are also discrepancies between expressed support and actual practice (Campbell, 2001). This could reflect professionals' perception of themselves as more supportive than users perceive them to be (Peck et al., 2002), resistance to the notion of sharing and transferring power to users or a clash of professionals' 'scientific' and users' more 'social' ways of thinking and working (Summers, 2003). The levels of partnership can be regarded through Tew et al.'s (2004) ladder of involvement which documents differing types of engagement (see Figure 2.1).

How have you been supported in your role?

Interview narratives

I'm not.

I'm fully supported.

Not really supported very well.

We are excellently supported.

As with the other questions earlier, the responses here revealed some very real differences of experience within the same organisation. It shows that we cannot become complacent and assume because some people are expressing very clearly and eloquently how happy they might be that this relates to everyone. Others may feel more reticent about voicing concerns for fear of becoming unpopular and losing future opportunities for involvement. Feeling properly supported involves having opportunities to build upon and consolidate one's educational input. Minogue and Handy (2010) found that service users' involvement was not equitable with some being invited for a single session whereas others having a much more sustained level of involvement. They recommend that for individuals to feel properly supported access needs to be more transparent and not just based on personal contact. This also considers periods of ill-health as

> people might not feel well at some point during what they're doing and for there to be another opportunity because everything then feels a failure. You need to be able to opt back in again when you're feeling a bit better.
>
> Minogue and Handy (2010, p. 20)

This was echoed by respondents who raised the worry around how to respond if feeling unwell and unable to fulfil one's obligations. Concerns here were of being dropped and not asked again to participate.

Further means of feeling supported included innovative approaches such being linked up with a learning mentor/buddy who could help clarify issues as well as highlight involvement opportunities. This could be investigated further as to the most effective background of mentors with perhaps an ideal choice being a fellow service user or carer.

Another interesting suggestion is the offering of non-monetary privileges such as library access. This appears to be a very pertinent suggestion and one which if we truly believe in partnership working should be facilitated. It is also worth considering in relation to those who do not request further payment because of the detrimental affect it would have upon their benefits.

CONCLUDING NOTE

This section highlights the depth and variety of service user involvement within healthcare education. It illustrates the mutual benefits that can be obtained by service users and learners and is certainly to be promoted. What is pertinent is the level and type of support provided by educational staff with a need to remain sensitive and aware of what it is we are asking service users to do. It is also important that service user inclusion does not become *tokenistic* but instead is a properly thought out and utilised source of expertise for learners and practitioners to benefit from.

REFERENCES

Alzheimer's Society. (2015). TalkingPoint Forum. www.alzheimers.org.uk, accessed 12 September, 2015.

Basset, T., Campbell, P. and Anderson, J. (2006). Service user/survivor involvement in mental health training and education: Overcoming the barriers. *Social Work Education.* 25(4), 393–402.

Bassman, R. (2000). Consumers/survivors/ex-patients as change facilitators. In F.J. Frese (Ed.), *The Role of Organized Psychology in Treatment of the Seriously Mentally Ill: New Directions for Mental Health Services* (pp. 93–102). Jossey Bass: San Francisco, CA.

Beresford, P. (2015). From 'other' to involved: User involvement in research: An emerging paradigm. *Nordic Social Work Research.* 3(2), 139–148.

Bipolar UK. (2015). e-community. http://www.bipolaruk.org.uk/, accessed 12 September, 2015.

Campbell, P. (2001). The role of users in psychiatric services in service development – Influence not power. *Psychiatric Bulletin.* 25, 87–88.

Clarke, S.P. and Holttum, S. (2013). Staff perspectives of service user involvement on two clinical psychology training courses. *Psychology Learning & Teaching.* 12(1), 32–43.

Crepaz-Keay, D. (2012). Evaluating service-user involvement in mental health services. In P. Ryan, S. Ramon and T. Greacen (Eds.), *Empowerment, Lifelong Learning and Recovery in Mental Health: Towards a New Paradigm* (pp. 146–153). Palgrave Macmillan: New York.

De Coster, I., Tambuyzer, E., Daem, R., Gouverneur, T., Cools, B., Verstraeten, J. and Van Audenhove, C. (2011). Towards expertise-by-experience in mental health care: Evaluation of a recovery-oriented training of (ex-) users of mental health care services. *Psychiatrische Praxis.* 38(S01). doi:10.1055/s-0031-1277809.

DoH (1990). NHS and Community Care Act. http://www.legislation.gov.uk, accessed 16 July, 2015.

DoH (1991). *The Patient's Charter.* HMSO: London, UK.

DoH (1994). Working in partnership: Report of the review of mental health nursing. HMSO: London, UK.

DoH (1995). *Building Bridges: A Guide to Arrangements for Inter-Agency Working for the Care and Protection of Severely Mentally Ill People.* HMSO: London, UK.

DoH (1999). *National Service Framework for Mental Health.* HMSO: London, UK.

DoH (2000). *The NHS Plan. A Plan for Investment, a Plan for Reform.* HMSO: London, UK.

DoH (2001a). The expert patient: A new approach to chronic disease management for the 21st century. http://webarchive.nationalarchives.gov.uk, accessed 16 July, 2015.

DoH (2001b). Mental health national service framework (and the NHS plan) workforce planning, education and training underpinning programme: Adult mental health services: Final report by the workforce action team. HMSO: London, UK.

DoH (2004). *NHS Improvement Plan.* HMSO: London, UK.

DoH (2005). *Mental Capacity Act.* HMSO: London, UK.

DoH (2009). *Living Well with Dementia: A National Dementia Strategy.* HMSO: London, UK.

DoH (2014). Achieving better access to mental health services by 2020. https://www.gov.uk, accessed 16 July, 2015.

El Enany, N., Currie, G. and Lockett, A. (2013). A paradox in healthcare service development: Professionalization of service users. *Social Science & Medicine.* 80, 24–30.

Higgins, A., Maguire, G., Watts, M., Creaner, M., Mccann, E., Rani, S. and Alexander, J. (2011). Service user involvement in mental health practitioner education in Ireland. *Journal of Psychiatric and Mental Health Nursing.* 18(6), 519–525.

Hitchen, S., Watkin, M., Williamson, G.R., Ambury, S., Bemrose, G., Cook, D. and Taylor, M. (2011). Lone voices have an emotional content: Focussing on mental health service user and carer involvement. *International Journal of Health Care Quality Assurance.* 24(2), 164–177.

Kemp, P. (2010). Introduction to mental health service user involvement. In J. Weinstein (Ed.), *Mental Health, Service User Involvement and Recovery* (pp. 15–29). Jessica Kingsley Publishers: London, UK.

Khoo, R., McVicar, A. and Brandon, D. (2004). Service user involvement in postgraduate mental health education. Does it benefit practice? *Journal of Mental Health.* 13(5), 481–492.

Lindow, V. (1999). Power, lies and injustice: The exclusion of service users' voices. In M. Parker (Ed.), *Ethics and Community in the Health Care Professions* (pp. 154–177). Routledge: London, UK.

McAndrew, S. and Samociuk, G. (2003). Reflecting together: Developing a new strategy for continuous user involvement in mental health nurse education. *Journal of Psychiatric and Mental Health Nursing.* 10, 616–621.

McKeown, M., Malihi-Shoja, L. and Downe, S. (2010). *Service User and Carer Involvement in Education for Health and Social Care.* Wiley Blackwell: Chichester, England.

McPhail, M. (2008). *Service User and Carer Involvement: Beyond Good Intentions.* Dunedin Academic Press: Edinburgh, Scotland.

Meehan, T. and Glover, H. (2007). Telling our story: Consumer perceptions of their role in mental health education. *Psychiatric Rehabilitation Journal.* 31(2), 152–154.

Mental Health Foundation (2003). *Surviving User-Led Research: Reflections on Supporting User-Led Research Projects.* Mental Health Foundation: London, UK.

Minogue, V., Boness, J., Brown, A. and Girdlestone, J. (2005). The impact of service user involvement in research. *International Journal of Health Care Quality Assurance.* 18(2), 103–112.

Minogue, V. and Handy, S. (2010). ALPS Research Capacity Final Report 3 of 3, Service user involvement in mental health training, education and research in West Yorkshire. University of Leeds: Leeds, England.

Minogue, V., Holt, B., Karban, K., Gelsthorpe, S., Firth, S. and Ramsay, T. (2009). User and carer involvement in mental health education, training and research – A literature review. *Mental Health and Learning Disabilities Research and Practice.* 6(2), 211–217.

Morgan, A. and Jones, D. (2009). Perceptions of service user and carer involvement in healthcare education and impact on students' knowledge and practice: A literature review. *Medical Teacher.* 31(2), 82–95.

NHS England (2013). Transforming participation in health and care. http://www.england.nhs.uk/, accessed 18 July, 2015.

NHS Management Executive (1992). *Local Voices: The Views of Local People in Purchasing for Health.* NHS Management Executive: Leeds, England.

NICE (2011). Care and support across all points on the care pathway. http://www.nice.org.uk, accessed 22 June, 2015.

Nickeas, R. (2007). The highs and lows of service user involvement. In T. Stickley and T. Basset (Eds.), *Teaching Mental Health* (pp. 35–42). John Wiley & Sons Ltd.: New York.

NMC (2010). Standards for pre-registration nursing education. http://www.nmc.org.uk.

NMC (2015). *The Code for Nurses and Midwives.* NMC: London, UK.

O'Donnell, H. and Gormley, K. (2013). Service user involvement in nurse education: Perceptions of mental health nursing students. *Journal of Psychiatric and Mental Health Nursing.* 20(3), 193–202.

Peck, E., Gulliver, P. and Towell, D. (2002). Information, consultation or control. User involvement in mental health services in England at the turn of the century. *Journal of Mental Health.* 11, 441–451.

Perry, J., Watkins, M., Gilbert, A. and Rawlinson, J. (2013). A systematic review of the evidence on service user involvement in interpersonal skills training of mental health students. *Journal of Psychiatric and Mental Health Nursing.* 20(6), 525–540.

Rhodes, C.A. and Nyawata, I. (2011). Service user and carer involvement in student nurse selection: Key stakeholder perspectives. *Nurse Education Today.* 31(5), 439–443.

Rush, B. (2008). Mental health service user involvement in nurse education: A catalyst for transformative learning. *Journal of Mental Health.* 17(5), 531–542.

Schneebeli, C., O'Brien, A., Lampshire, D. and Hamer, H. (2010). Service user involvement in undergraduate mental health nursing in New Zealand. *International Journal of Mental Health Nursing.* 19(1), 30–35.

Simons, L., Tee, S., Lathlean, J., Burgess, A., Herbert, L. and Gibson, C. (2007). A socially inclusive approach to user participation in Higher Education. *Journal of Advanced Nursing.* 58(3), 246–255.

Speed, S., Griffiths, J., Horne, M. and Keeley, P. (2012). Pitfalls, perils and payments: Service user, carers and teaching staff perceptions of the barriers to involvement in nursing education. *Nurse Education Today.* 32(7), 829–834.

Spiers, S., Harney, K. and Chilvers, G. (2005). Service user involvement in forensic mental health: Can it work? *Journal of Forensic Psychiatry & Psychology.* 16(2), 211–220.

Summers, A. (2003). Involving users in the development of mental health services: A study of psychiatrists' views. *Journal of Mental Health.* 12, 161–174.

Tait, L. and Lester, H. (2005). Encouraging user involvement in mental health services. *Advances in Psychiatric Treatment.* 11, 168–175.

Tew, J., Gell, C. and Foster, F. (2004). *A Good Practice Guide. Learning from Experience.* Involving service users and carers in mental health education and training. Mental Health in Higher Education. NIMH: Nottingham, England.

The Mid Staffordshire NHS Foundation Trust Public Inquiry (2013). Report of the Mid Staffordshire NHS Foundation Trust Public Inquiry: Executive summary. Stationery Office: London, UK.

Turner, M. and Beresford, P. (2005). *Contributing on Equal Terms: Service User Involvement and the Benefit System.* Social Care Institute for Excellence: London, UK.

Weinstein, J. (2010). *Mental Health, Service User Involvement and Recovery. Mental Health, Service User Involvement and Recovery.* Jessica Kingsley Publishers: London, UK.

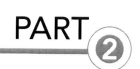

PART ②

THE LIVED EXPERIENCE IN MENTAL HEALTH

'Standing on a cliff edge'
Living with anxiety

INTRODUCTION

This chapter explores the multi-faceted range of experiences concerned with *anxiety*. Whilst at certain levels causing significant distress for people it can at the other end of the spectrum be regarded as a 'normal' reaction to situations in which people find themselves. This provides a beneficial, protective function alerting one of danger as well as helping to focus attention and improve performance. We can all relate to the experience of anxiety although to very different degrees of emotional intensity. Mild to moderate levels of anxiety are part of most people's lives and generally coped well with. More severe levels though can be debilitating and impact upon all aspects of a person's life including work, education, leisure pursuits and relationships. The physical and psychological effects (see Figure 3.1) can create a difficult and pervasive spiral of negative thinking. Being unable to find relief for one's concerns can cause a person much distress and influence ways of responding to situations. Concentration, attention, motivation and drive can all be severely decreased, making all of these aspects problematic, frustrating and at times agonising. Areas such as sleep can be strongly impacted upon further heightening a person's levels of stress and agitation. Without proper support (and in some cases even with support) anxiety problems can take over people's lives and leave them feeling 'different', helpless, impotent, vulnerable, stressed and fearful. Personal means of coping with this can include avoidance, isolating oneself or seeking support from drink and drugs. Such coping methods in turn cause their own problems and can develop into a downward spiral, heightening a person's sense of difference, lowered confidence and feelings of helplessness. These issues will be examined within this chapter which is concerned with what it feels like to experience problems with anxiety, ways in which different types of support are experienced and aspects relating to living well and coping.

Briefly consider situations that make you fearful or uneasy.

How would you feel if you were unable to get respite from these feelings?

Physical effects

Short-term effects

- Increased muscular tension – discomfort and headaches
- Rapid breathing – light-headed, shaky, pins and needles
- Rising blood pressure – pounding heart
- Changes in the blood supply to digestive system – nausea and sickness
- Urgent need to visit the toilet
- 'Butterflies' in your stomach

Long-term effects

- Fear, tension and lack of sleep – lowered resistance to infection
- Digestive difficulties
- Depression

Psychological effects

More fearful, alert, on edge, irritable and unable to relax or concentrate

Overwhelming desire to seek reassurance of others, to be weepy and dependent

Thinking affected – fear the worst is going to happen, seeing everything negatively and becoming pessimistic

Figure 3.1 Anxiety (physical and psychological effects).

SECTION 1: EXPERIENCING ANXIETY

Interview narratives

It's every day, it's every single day … There's never a day that goes by when it doesn't affect me.

It dominates my life really … it prevents me doing a lot of things and gives me lots of very scary symptoms.

I get very jittery, on edge, feel as though I'm going to have some sort of brain haemorrhage … or a pain in my chest and I think I'm going to die of a heart attack.

I just isolated myself and cut off from friends.

It was as if there was no hope and there was this intense fear that something had gone badly wrong.

Anxiety has had a big impact on my life … as a result of it I got depression.

I remember the GP appointment. It was only a 10 minute walk away but I could barely walk without getting out of breath so I started thinking it was something even more serious.

I can't show somebody else the experience or make them come into my body to actually feel what it's like.

Drink was a great way of coping … until it actually stopped working.

The varied manifestations of anxiety disorder examined within this chapter incorporate those categorised by the *DSM-V* (American Psychiatric Association, 2013) but have been widened to also focus upon obsessive–compulsive disorder (OCD) and post-traumatic stress disorder (PTSD). Those featured include

- Phobias
- Social anxiety disorder (SAD)
- Panic disorder
- Generalised anxiety disorder (GAD)
- OCD
- PTSD

This list could be extended to incorporate other problems such as body dysmorphic disorder, hoarding disorder, trichotillomania (hair pulling disorder) and excoriation (skin picking disorder) although because of the limited space within this chapter, the main emphasis will be upon the more commonly experienced anxiety-related disorders listed earlier.

PHOBIAS

A phobia is an extreme form of fear or anxiety triggered by a particular situation or object even when there is no actual danger. A fear becomes a phobia if it lasts for more than 6 months and has a significant impact on how a person lives their day-to-day life (Mind, 2013a). Phobias can be categorised as specific phobia or agoraphobia. A specific phobia involves a strong fear and avoidance of one particular object or situation, where direct exposure may elicit a panic attack. Whilst agoraphobia relates to a fear of open spaces, the essence concerns a fear of panic attacks and being in situations from which escape might be difficult (Bourne, 2011). There are many different types of specific phobia with more than 300 reported from the familiar to the less familiar (Buchanan and Coulson, 2012). Symptoms of a phobia can be seen in Figure 3.2.

With some phobias, the focal point for a person's fear can be encountered through many different experiences and can greatly impact upon all spheres of their life. An example here can be seen with a Time to Change (2013a) blogger's emetophobia (fear of vomiting):

> As I grew up, I knew there was a problem. I couldn't watch any medical programmes on TV without having to cover up my eyes, I stayed away from people who said they were feeling poorly and I was constantly worried that I was going to be ill too. I don't drink alcohol either. Friends joke around and call me 'boring' at times but the thought of getting ill from alcohol petrifies me.

This phobia greatly restricted her ability to travel, socialise and go out for meals. It also made it hard for her to talk with others about her problems for fear of being judged or ridiculed. She viewed medication with uncertainty on account of one of the listed side effects – 'nausea'. Her experience illustrates the all-encompassing impact that a phobia can have upon a person's daily life. It also highlights the acute sense a person may have of feeling *different*, weak or vulnerable. There is also a significant degree of reliance

Physical symptoms

- Feeling unsteady, dizzy, light-headed or faint
- Feeling like you are choking
- A pounding heart, palpitations or accelerated heart rate
- Chest pain or tightness in the chest
- Sweating
- Hot or cold flushes
- Shortness of breath or a smothering sensation
- Nausea, vomiting or diarrhoea
- Numbness or tingling sensations
- Trembling or shaking

Other symptoms

- Feeling out of touch with reality or detached from your body
- Fear of fainting
- Fear of losing control
- Fear of dying

Figure 3.2 Symptoms of a phobia.

indicated upon the support, sensitivity and understanding of other people in order to maintain activities and relationships. The vulnerability to ridicule or teasing is illustrated by a young concerning her fear of pigeons (Phobia Fear Release, 2014). She recounts a distressing experience at school encountering a pigeon in the toilets and having to run away to escape, shutting herself away in a cubicle to try and cope with her feelings of anxiety and embarrassment. This is an upsetting and unsettling experience but one which potentially can be met by less than supportive responses from peers, being made fun of and teased for what may be seen of as a 'silly' and insignificant fear. The main issue for those experiencing phobias is that they are no laughing matter. They can be totally debilitating, deeply distressing and impacting detrimentally upon all spheres of a person's life.

SOCIAL ANXIETY DISORDER

SAD is the most common anxiety disorder with an early age of onset and is a risk factor for subsequent depressive illness and substance abuse (Stein and Stein, 2008). A diagnosis of SAD is made in connection with persistent symptoms lasting for a period of 6 months or more. It is considerably disabling, causes significant distress and interferes with a person's ordinary routine in social settings (American Psychiatric Association, 2013). It is one of the most common of the anxiety disorders and relates to a persistent fear in social situations, out of proportion to the actual threat posed. Typical situations that might be anxiety-provoking include meeting people, public speaking, starting conversations and being seen in public. Whilst these can be commonly experienced concerns, those with SAD worry excessively about them, before, during and after situations. The fears include saying or doing something which might be perceived as humiliating or embarrassing such as blushing, sweating, shaking, looking anxious or appearing incompetent (NICE, 2013). A Time to Change (2014a) blogger recalls his terror when having to speak in front of others making him feel physically sick:

I have used all my powers and energies keeping up the pretence that I was OK, when all the time I would be crying out inside. I have felt ashamed, weak and worthless that I have been saddled with these mental health illnesses. At times I think I would happily trade my depression and anxiety for cancer. At least that way I could talk openly about it, nay shout it from the roof tops, without the fear of stigma from friends and work colleagues.

This is an extremely powerful expression illustrating how the depth of a person's anxiety can far transcend the 'normal' ranges of trepidation and discomfort felt. Here, there is a very real sense of agony and shame as well as helplessness at being so incapacitated. The associated stigma only adds to the distress felt and difficulty in seeking help. The statement about trading anxiety problems with that of cancer is a startling one and strongly underlines the depth to which discrimination can be felt. The feeling of weakness and powerlessness is a pervasive emotion connected with anxiety disorders. It highlights the feeling that one should be able to cope with one's problems and that the inability to do so is a sign of weakness. Thoughts about potential responses from others of 'pull yourself together' and 'stop worrying' only serve to maintain feelings of weakness and lessen the inclination to talk with others. Turk et al. (2008) state that as a large number of people in the population are shy and inhibited, problems encountered with SAD are liable to being regarded merely as common traits not requiring specialist interventions. Fortunately there is a more sophisticated appreciation now of SAD and its prevalence, chronic and pernicious nature, and neurobiological underpinnings.

> In what ways do you feel a person experiencing SAD might be limited in their life? How might this make them feel?

PANIC DISORDER

According to the *DSM-V* (American Psychiatric Association, 2013), a panic attack is an abrupt surge of intense fear or intense discomfort that reaches a peak within minutes. This can occur from either a calm or anxious state with over three of the following symptoms occurring:

- Palpitations, pounding heart, or accelerated heart rate
- Sweating
- Trembling or shaking
- Sensations of shortness of breath or smothering
- Feelings of choking
- Chest pain or discomfort
- Nausea or abdominal distress
- Feeling dizzy, unsteady, light-headed or faint
- Chills or heat sensations
- Paraesthesias (numbness or tingling sensations)
- Derealisation (feelings of unreality)/depersonalisation (detached from oneself)

- Fear of losing control or 'going crazy'
- Fear of dying

Intense panic can last for a few minutes but can return in waves and last for up to 2 hours (Bourne, 2011). Looking at these symptoms it is not surprising that a person in the midst of a panic attack can strongly believe that they are having a heart attack. As the actress Stephane Cole recounted:

> Did I think I was going to die? When the panic attacks were bad yes.
>
> Gekoski and Broome (2014, p. 75)

This will evidently serve to heighten a person's feelings of panic and distress and strongly influence a person's avoidant behaviour, finding means of distancing oneself from situations that are seen as panic-inducing. It can be very restrictive and socially isolating as reflected by McLean (2014) who suffered for years with a panic disorder. She arduously disguised her panic attacks finding excuses for avoiding situations and not attending functions. These avoidant strategies were ineffective though in preventing the build-up of panic attacks which she remembers occurring anywhere, even if alone watching TV or carrying out domestic chores as mundanely routine as washing up. A blogger relates the impact that her experience of panic had upon her:

> I was sat in a hot, sweaty lecture theatre when suddenly I felt like I needed to escape. I then went through the toughest time in my life. I was unable to eat, I hardly left my flat and I found it hard to go to lectures or even go on nights out.
>
> Time to Change (2014b)

She also detailed the sense of difference felt with her anxiety stripping away her ability to function 'normally', something her friends, classmates and family appeared to be able to easily do. Karen (ADAA, 2014a) recalls being rushed to the hospital after her first panic attack:

> I was released with a diagnosis of panic disorder, which ran in my family. Then I got worse, and I pretty much became afraid of my own shadow. I also had burning sensations in my chest, weakness all over, and I felt so fatigued I couldn't even stand. My anxiety was so terrible I couldn't eat; I just shook … Depression set in and I got worse.

This narrative illustrates the intensity of feelings and symptoms which are experienced physically as well as psychologically. They can appear very quickly, leaving the person in severe distress and unable to cope.

GENERALISED ANXIETY DISORDER

GAD is a persistent and common disorder with an unfocused worry not connected to recent stressful events, although aggravated by certain situations (NICE, 2011). It is characterised by feelings of threat, restlessness, irritability, sleep disturbance, tension and symptoms such as palpitations, dry mouth and sweating (Tyrer and Baldwin, 2006). It is estimated that GAD affects between 1% and 5% of the general population (Gale and Davidson, 2007). The severity of symptoms with GAD varies from person to person with some people experiencing only one or two symptoms, while others have many more. GAD is diagnosed when a person worries excessively about a variety of everyday problems for at least 6 months (National Institute of Mental Health, 2015). Like other anxiety disorders, GAD is often chronic if untreated and is associated with substantial disability equivalent to other chronic physical health problems such as arthritis and diabetes (Kendall et al., 2011). A distinction from other anxiety disorders is that those affected with GAD may not know what they are feeling anxious about. Being unaware of the triggers can intensify a person's sense of unease and anxiety with the worry that a solution will not be able to be found (NHS Choices, 2014a). Melanie Higgins (ADAA, 2014b) recalls having flashes of fear and of feeling sick whenever people around her were unwell:

> These incidents were brief, but I knew they weren't normal. I started to worry more about my family becoming sick. I recognized that my fear was irrational and this concerned me. One October day my husband reported that he had an upset stomach. I was completely overcome with fear, worry, and anxiety. I felt sick to my stomach and couldn't eat.

Josh Lewin (ADAA, 2014c) describes how GAD influenced his thoughts and actions:

> I began to stay away from parties. When I did go and fake my way through, I would usually leave upset, gripped by the weight of having been such a fraud. At my lowest moments, everything and everyone in the world was a threat. In an anxious state, all I could see were the things I couldn't do or didn't have, and people I couldn't be. I had no appreciation whatsoever of anything I already was. No matter what I did, the foreboding sense was that it would never be enough … I'd be racked with guilt about things I'd done poorly and trembling with worry that I'd soon screw something else up too.

The essence being recounted here is the fear of not being good enough and being vulnerable to making mistakes and failing. It can develop into a self-perpetuating cycle with anxieties and worries placing attention upon the detection and interpretation of potential threats, causing more distress and exacerbating feelings of being out of control (Waters and Craske, 2005).

Obsessive–Compulsive Disorder

OCD differs from other anxiety disorders such as phobias in that the stimulus provoking the unease is internally driven. It is, as Veale and Willson (2011) assert, essentially a problem of trying too hard to reduce the threat of harm. There is a high co-morbidity rate between OCD and depression as well as anorexia nervosa with many symptoms in common (Kaye et al., 2004; Swinbourne and Touyz, 2007). People with OCD often feel they have a pivotal responsibility for either preventing or causing harm and the following of a

---

The more you

- Check something, the more responsible you'll feel.
- Check something, the more doubts you'll have.
- Try to neutralise or support a thought or image, the more intrusive it will become.
- Analyse a thought, the more significant it will become in your mind.
- Try to reduce threats, the more aware of them you will become.
- Try to reassure yourself or get reassurance from others, the more your doubts return.
- Wash, the more likely you are to feel dirty and to wash again.
- Avoid something, the more your fear of it will increase.

Figure 3.3 Compulsions. (From Veale, D. and Willson, R., eds., *Taking Control of OCD: Inspirational Stories of Hope and Recovery*, Robinson: London, UK, 2011.)

compulsion. As illustrated in Figure 3.3, the following of compulsions serves to reinforce the sense of uncertainty and tension a person has.

According to the *DSM-V* (American Psychiatric Association, 2013), obsessions are defined by

- Recurrent and persistent thoughts, urges or images (intrusive and unwanted) that cause marked anxiety or distress. The individual attempts to ignore or suppress them with some other thought or action (i.e. by performing a compulsion).

Whilst compulsions are defined by

- Repetitive behaviours (e.g. handwashing, ordering and checking) or mental acts (e.g. praying, counting and repeating words silently) that the individual feels driven to perform in response to an obsession.
- The behaviours or mental acts aimed at preventing or reducing anxiety, distress or some dreaded event or situation.

A blogger *recounts her problems with repeated handwashing* and a preoccupation with numbers and rituals with which she had no control over:

> I came to realise my obsessional thoughts were irrational, but that did not lessen the impulse to relieve the acute anxiety by performing compulsive behaviours, as well as mental rituals to 'prevent harm' happening to me or, more often than not, someone I cared about. Attempting to resist the compulsions resulted in such an overwhelming feeling of anxiety and dread, I felt like I was standing on a cliff edge. I'd break out into a sweat, I'd feel sick and I would shake.
>
> Time to Change (2014c)

This narrative illustrates just how agonisingly stuck people can be with their compulsive behaviours. If prevented from completing rituals the person can feel a sense of helpless dread and panic, preoccupied with obsessional thoughts. This in some cases involves elaborate or very arduous steps to resume and complete rituals. Joe Wells (2006) recounts the time-consuming and difficult nature in restarting very intricate and lengthy numerical patterns which involved tapping various objects. These experiences can affect anybody, irrespective of status, causing distress, influencing responses and imposing severe restrictions upon their lives.

How would you feel if experiencing some of the thoughts and compulsions addressed here?

POST-TRAUMATIC STRESS DISORDER

PTSD is an anxiety disorder caused by very traumatic, frightening or distressing events which include serious road accidents, violent personal assaults, sexual abuse, military combat, terrorist attacks and natural disasters. It can develop immediately after experiencing such an event or some time later, even after a period of years. A person with PTSD will often relive the traumatic event through nightmares and flashbacks, and may experience feelings of isolation, irritability and guilt. They may also have problems sleeping and find concentrating difficult (NHS Choices, 2013). These symptoms (see Figure 3.4) are often severe and persistent enough to have a debilitating impact upon the person's day-to-day life. Simon, an ex-serviceman, developed PTSD symptoms following his traumatic Bosnian war experience which included sleep disturbances, flashbacks, severe anxiety and memory problems (Your Stories, 2012a). He felt unable to reveal his emotions to others with the worry that this would be seen as a sign of weakness. Abusing alcohol provided him with a temporary means of escaping from what he was feeling although subsequently producing further problems.

Re-experiencing symptoms

- Flashbacks – reliving the trauma (including physical symptoms, racing heart/sweating)
- Bad dreams
- Frightening thoughts

Avoidance symptoms

- Staying away from places, events or objects (reminders of the experience)
- Feeling emotionally numb
- Feeling strong guilt, depression or worry
- Losing interest in activities that were enjoyable in the past
- Having trouble remembering the dangerous event

Hyperarousal symptoms

- Being easily startled
- Feeling tense or 'on edge'
- Having difficulty sleeping and/or having angry outbursts

Figure 3.4 Post-traumatic stress disorder signs and symptoms. (From National Institute of Mental Health, 2015, http://www.nimh.nih.gov.)

Philips' (ADAA, 2014d) blog illustrates the impact that a series of traumatic experiences had upon him:

> My PTSD was triggered by several traumas, including a childhood laced with physical, mental, and sexual abuse, as well as an attack at knifepoint that left me thinking I would die. I would never be the same after that attack. For me there was no safe place in the world, not even my home … For months after the attack, I couldn't close my eyes without envisioning the face of my attacker. I suffered horrific flashbacks and nightmares. For four years after the attack I was unable to sleep alone in my house. I obsessively checked windows, doors, and locks.

This experience highlights the pervasive feelings of threat and inability a person has of feeling safe in any environment. As Hapke et al. (2006) state, the type of traumatic events play a crucial role with rape, sexual assaults and other personal assaults being associated with a higher risk of PTSD compared to less personally traumatic events such as serious accidents. It needs acknowledging though that these experiences will vary in terms of impact and intensity for each person.

DIAGNOSIS

How would you feel if diagnosed with an anxiety disorder?

What would your immediate support needs be?

The receipt of a diagnosis, as with other mental health problems, can evoke extremely polarised feelings, for example, relief and reassurance or shame and concern. To understand how a diagnosis can be experienced with feelings of relief it is worth considering how desperate and difficult the time pre-diagnosis can be. McLean (2014) relates how she suffered for years with a panic disorder, feeling totally exhausted in both body and mind from being in a constant state of overdrive. The strain of living with this condition and pretending to others that things were OK led to her experiencing suicidal thoughts. The receipt of a diagnosis was the first step in tackling her problems and rebuilding her life. A similar experience is recounted by Andy (Mind, 2013b) who initially attributed the panic attacks he was experiencing to overwork, stress and changing personal circumstances. He struggled to remain in control and feared being 'found out' and evoking responses of ridicule or pity. Getting a diagnosis and bringing his problems out into the open felt hugely welcome, as efforts could then focus upon much needed rest and recovery. A Time to Change (2012a) blogger reflected that seeing the words OCD on the referral form was a great relief:

> It was a recognised illness that was treatable. It was no longer something that maybe only I had. This meant I was normal!

This reflects a sense of hope as well as the feeling of not being alone, something reflected by a narrator in Veale and Willson's (2011, p. 7) text:

> Following the diagnosis, I was so elated that it wasn't just me who had this problem, and that having it didn't necessarily guarantee that I would one day feature on Crimewatch.

There are some important aspects being related here concerning the *naming* of what may have been formerly experienced as a confusing and incomprehensible collection of symptoms. A diagnosis provides a vital point of reference, not only for those experiencing symptoms but also for others around them. There can also be a sense of connection fostered with other people who are experiencing similar issues. This can be contrasted though by experiences where the receipt of a diagnosis feels scary and intimidating:

> OCD is like the bad guy in Harry Potter: we don't even want to mention its name.

> Wells (2006, p. 96)

It is important to note the changing nature of one's emotions and thoughts about what having a diagnosis means. Whilst Kant (2008) initially expressed being happy with his diagnosis and having a name to clarify what he was going through, he later recalled feeling angry, depressed and more anxious with the contemplation of having a condition without a quick fix. The process which individuals go through before getting a diagnosis related to an anxiety disorder can be far from satisfactory as reported by a number of Social Anxiety UK (SAUK) members. Postings reflect experiences of receiving no diagnosis at all, only being given vague references at best, or being diagnosed after the duration of many years of suffering. There are also a number of statements about the experience of initially being diagnosed with other conditions such as depression. This problem was identified by Stein et al. (2012) in that where a co-existing depression was present anxiety disorders may not be detected. Another discussion forum concerning anxiety problems can be found on the Patient site with postings illustrative of the many unanswered questions which individuals feel have not been covered by their GP. There are many statements about the limited time slot offered, scant space for all the questions people have as well as a lack of understanding as to what has been said about one's diagnosis and related treatment options.

TRIVIALISATION AND LACK OF UNDERSTANDING

A particular problem encountered concerns the lack of understanding that many people have about the reality of living with anxiety disorders. Personal narratives reflect upon frequent instances of feeling dismissed, trivialised or make fun of with what is experienced as very real distress. It appears that anxiety disorders are frequently misconceived or regarded through stereotypical notions as to what is involved. This is encountered within one's social sphere, the media or society in general. It causes real distress and frustration to those concerned, feeling that problems are not being taken seriously.

This is commonly experienced by those living with OCD as reflected through a number of personal narratives shared on the Time to Change website:

> I'm always sad and frustrated to see OCD trivialised because it can be all-consuming and leave you with no quality of life. All we seem to get from the media is the caricaturing and parody of a serious illness.

Time to Change (2014c)

It was also felt that OCD is a massively misunderstood condition:

> Just go and search twitter right now for 'ocd' to find proof and find hundreds of people 'so wishing I had OCD #likeclean' or 'aaah I'm so OCD about my iTunes!!'. These people do not realise how serious the condition is, all they know is what TV, celebrities or pop culture tells them...I had many friends say to me 'I saw that show [Obsessive Compulsive Cleaners] about your condition last night, you can come clean my flat anytime mate!'

Time to Change (2013b)

This blogger further relates that what the media predominantly focus upon are the compulsive behaviours that people exhibit to the detriment of:

> The horrific panic, stunning fear and immense trauma obsessive compulsive disorder gives its sufferers.

It seems that the part which is of most interest to media groups are the elements which make their products more appealing, dramatic or entertaining, thereby stimulating commercial interest. The lack of sensitivity and attention to what is being experienced is also reflected by a blogger *who finds very* wearisome the fact that people commonly regard OCD as being exclusively a problem with handwashing or tidying things which does not at all appreciate what she is struggling with:

> My head is like a horrible person, picking up on all the negative feelings I have about myself and obsessively bombarding me with them. I am told how rubbish I am, how sad, how nobody wants anything to do with me and that I will never be 'normal', whatever that means. This isn't a voice in my head, it's me telling me, which is why it is nearly impossible to fight. I compulsively pick away at myself, I question everything and if I can see the negative in something then I do.

Time to Change (2013c)

The SAUK (2014) discussion forum includes a number of discussion threads relating to how members react to commonly heard statements such as 'quieten down' or 'he never shuts up' in relation to their withdrawn and reticent behaviour. There was a wide range of opinion given with a number of people regarding it as 'harmless banter' or attempts by others to draw them into conversation. For other people though it was felt as hurtful, insensitive and dismissive. It can be especially upsetting where pranks or jokes are played in a thoughtless manner. Melissa North's experience concerning her fear of cheese is illustrative of the general lack of comprehension from others about what it is like to have a phobia:

> I came back from a full day studying to find cheese smudged all over my door. A flatmate had found it funny to graffiti on my bedroom door and I just couldn't go near it. That wasn't even the worst part, they left a trail of cheese outside my door so there was no way I could go in … My friends and family think it's hilarious but it's really awful. I hate going near the stuff, and seeing people eat it is horrendous.

Daily Mail (2014)

Even the newspaper reporting her experience could not resist joking at her expense with their headline:

> She must Brie terrified.

The lack of sensitivity and awareness of what a person might be experiencing internally and the impact upon a person who is made fun of is summed up by a blogger on the OCD UK site (2014) who highlights how painful it is being laughed at concerning an experience which can destroy people's lives. This narrative goes on to stress that what is needed instead of being made fun of is understanding.

Whilst more-commonly shared fears (e.g. spiders) might be easier to acknowledge, other less-experienced ones can be hard to appreciate leading in instances of the person being teased, made fun of or rejected. When considered from the viewpoint of the person with anxiety the behaviour of others can be regarded as hurtful, bullying and dismissive. Yet from the opposite perspective, the person with anxiety might be thought of as 'silly' or 'childish'. A glance at the list of phobic stimuli in Figure 3.5 may illustrate this point with some selected examples which others might find hard to relate to as feared objects. These have been deliberately chosen and feature elements which could be seen as comical yet for the person experiencing fear induce very real distress. The lack of understanding from others can be extremely upsetting as illustrated by a Time to Change (2013d) blogger who is agoraphobic. She recounts the humiliation and shame she felt by the dismissive and insensitive attitude of the bank employee who insisted she come to the branch despite being informed that it would be impossible.

What are your feelings about the types of phobia listed in Figure 3.5?

How would you feel in relation to other people if affected by any of these?

Ailurophobia – fear of cats
Alektorophobia – fear of chickens
Alliumphobia – fear of garlic
Aulophobia – fear of flutes
Botanophobia – fear of plants
Chaetophobia – fear of hair
Chronomentrophobia – fear of clocks
Coulrophobia – fear of clowns
Geniophobia – fear of chins
Koumpounophobia – fear of buttons
Lachanophobia – fear of vegetables
Omphalophobia – fear of belly buttons
Papyrophobia – fear of paper
Peladophobia – fear of bald people
Pogonophobia – fear of beards
Pupaphobia – fear of puppets
Symmetrophobia – fear of symmetry

Figure 3.5 Types of phobia.

SHARING EXPERIENCE

What makes living with anxiety disorders particularly isolating and alienating is the difficulty in sharing one's experience with others. Concerns about others knowing about one's problems include the fear of being teased, dismissed or humiliated. A Time to Change (2012b) blogger relates her experience:

> I've never really felt like this is something one should share too openly for fear of being regarded as 'crazy'. If I tell people, I think to myself, 'that makes me different', and not different in a cool way. But different in an 'uh-oh, mental alert' kind of way.

She also relates the associated misconception and stereotypical notions around OCD as causing problems:

> There's been many a comical moment when, on disclosing OCD to friends, they've commented on my untidy room or the number of mugs that lie around unwashed for days … it's made explaining my OCD even harder because I feel like I don't 'fit the bill'.

This type of response can feel insulting and hurtful. A Time to Change (2013e) blogger recalls revealing her anxiety problems to her employer and not having this kept in confidence. Her subsequent experience was of feeling excluded by colleagues, sensing that people were whispering about her and staring at her. *The result of this was feeling more reluctant within future work environments in sharing her difficulties with others. This has a strong impact of leaving people feeling very much alone with their experiences and unsure as to the safety of talking about them with others. There can also be the fear that others, even close family and friends, simply would not be able to understand.* Former model Jemma Kidd (O'Brien, 2011) recalls:

> I was in my bedroom when the full-blown attack came on…The most unnerving thing was that there had been no trigger – nothing awful had happened. And I felt I couldn't tell anyone – in my family, everyone was always so together and I thought no one would understand.

This highlights the strong sense of separateness, disconnectedness and detachment which can be felt. As Damien (Mind, 2014) observes the most stressful and anxiety provoking experiences

> tend to be the ones involving the most people, yet to suffer anxiety is to feel that you're totally alone, in a cold stark world where no one else can reach you.

This is particularly experienced with social anxiety and many SAUK members share how excruciatingly hard it feels, desperately wanting to socialise yet feeling powerless and unable to do so. Their postings include feeling paralysed through worries about what to say, fears about what others might think, convictions about being regarded as boring and the sense that they would not be liked. A core feeling was that of loneliness and the concern over always being alone. Watching others socialising, laughing and having fun was the cause of much sadness and pain. This is a terribly distressing experience and highlights something of the depth to which a person's sense of despair can be experienced. The sense of alienation and need for connectedness can be lessened through identification with others, even with remote figures such as celebrities. Kant (2008), disconnected from others through his experiences with anxiety, recounts finding solace in famous people he could relate to such as Marilyn Manson.

> If you had a problem with anxiety,
>
> Who could you talk to about it and why?
>
> Who would you feel reluctant to talk with and why?

CONCEALMENT

As well as feeling unable to talk with others about one's difficulties, individuals experiencing anxiety problems can attempt to conceal what they experience for fear of negative or critical responses (Corrigan et al., 2009). Bretécher (2013) describes how she hid her OCD because:

> I was repulsed and desperately ashamed of these thoughts, and terrified that if I told anyone I'd get arrested. So I kept them quiet, and fought them in lots of tiny, secret ways.

This was influenced through worries about being disbelieved, regarded as *freakish* and rejected. She feared people's reactions if disclosing and thought others would not believe her, reject her, be disgusted with her or think she was a freak. It can leave individuals feeling very isolated and obstruct opportunities for seeking support. There can be a strongly associated sense of shame at having experiences or thoughts which one regards as 'abnormal'. Fears around stigma and rejection can lead to attempts to conceal or 'normalise' one's behaviour with others (Fennell and Liberato, 2007). An example of this can be seen with Wells' (2006) compulsive tapping behaviour which he attempted to camouflage when having to repeat a ritual through pretending he had forgotten something. It only though provided limited relief and as Wells (2006) noted can delay opportunities to seek help.

PREOCCUPATION

The nature of one's thoughts and fears with anxiety disorders can be very intense and all encompassing. The sense of preoccupation can be exhausting and draining, leaving little space for rest or relief. Annie (Mind, 2013c) reports the excruciating experience of being unable to sleep, night after night, 'pleading' with her brain for a few hours respite, waking each morning feeling drained, irritable and lethargic. It is also worth considering the emotional toll that thoughts can have upon a person which can seem relenting and torturous. Millwallant (2013) writes about the disturbing impulses he has experienced about harming himself or others. This was a relentlessly distressing experience leading him to withdraw and isolate himself from others. A narrative on the Time to Change site relates:

> My obsessions are mainly focused on the people I love the most: the idea that I have the 'power' to stop harm or even death coming to them is a huge weight to carry.
>
> Time to Change (2014d)

This led to certain protective rituals being created, having to touch a wall a number of times in order to prevent calamitous events occurring. This was a draining and terrifying process. The issue here concerns the potency with which thoughts and feelings about anxiety can be associated. This can be regarded within the Gestalt (King and Wertheimer, 2007) concept of *figure and ground* whereby certain perceptual stimuli are focused upon with other aspects relegated to the background. Here, elements connected with anxious thoughts are given greater prominence to other more rational or measured ones making it hard to view things with a more balanced context. Objects or situations which do not pose actual risk of danger can be perceived as threatening and harmful. Attention can be primarily related to the distressing nature of one's thoughts or the seeking of strategies or approaches to gain some relief.

It is unsurprising given the distress and disruption caused to one's life that depression features significantly for those experiencing anxiety problems. Indeed, over 75% of those experiencing OCD also experienced depression with roughly 30% diagnosed with the co-morbidity of major depression (Masellis et al., 2003). Aspects covered earlier relating to different anxiety problems highlight feelings of being different, isolated and ridiculed. The preoccupation with distressing thoughts and feelings can allow little respite and be emotionally and physically draining. This illustrates the need to acknowledge the impact anxiety problems can have upon a person and gear supportive interventions accordingly.

Seeking reassurance

What do you think is experienced by people with anxiety when seeking reassurance?

Struggling with painful and distressing experiences will naturally create a desire to seek consolation and support from others. This relates to feelings of security, acknowledgement and acceptance. The potency of one's patterns of thinking or preoccupation with anxious or unsettling thoughts makes it hard to actually feel *reassured*. Therefore, the consistency or repetitiveness of one's requests for help can be viewed negatively as 'attention seeking', 'demanding' or 'clingy' behaviour. The less than favourable responses or irritated manner of those consulted will reinforce negative thinking patterns and in turn create the need for further reassurance to be sought. The problem here is when it does not work or only provide momentary relief. Discussion threads on the OCD UK (2015) forum show recognition that reassurance can be counterproductive and advise against giving this excessively to each other. Attempts to resist reassurance seeking can be very difficult:

> I can see that my partner and everyone is sick and tired of it yet I keep on with it [seeking reassurance].

> OCD Action (2008)

The act or compulsion to seek reassurance can feel addictive and difficult to resist because of one's inability to tolerate feelings of discomfort or uncertainty experienced. It can however act as a reinforcement providing the message that anxiety-related thoughts or fears are significant (OCDLA, 2010). The repeated postings and pleas for help seen in discussion forums (Why is nobody responding – Anxiety Forum) show clearly that for some people difficulties are not being resolved through others' responses. A study by Clerkin et al. (2014) examined the interpersonal effects of reassurance seeking in the social networking site Facebook. They found many individuals to be ineffective in their communication strategies with a resultant increase in feelings of not belonging or being a burden. This in turn can strengthen the need for the seeking of reassurance. There are however very real needs which are going unmet here, and supportive interventions are required which address a person's internal core feelings driving this need for reassurance.

Maladaptive coping methods

The experience of feeling out of control is particularly felt with anxiety problems. Attempts to deal with symptoms and self-treat anxiety cover a range of approaches, a number of which only provide temporary respite. These include seeking reassurance or self-medicating through alcohol and drugs. In order to cope with the distressing effects of anxiety a person can feel tempted to seek relief through drinking or taking drugs which can help to alleviate the intensity of one's distress (Mind, 2013a). Other self-medicating substances utilised by those with anxiety problems include tobacco, although smoking has been found to increase the risk of panic disorder (Isensee et al., 2003).

Rich Hilson (Your Stories, 2012b) describes drinking as a means of coping with many years of depression and anxiety:

> I began to realise that alcohol was a problem for me; I would drink all weekend but was in denial that it affected my state of mind.

This is where this particular approach to coping creates its own problems for those concerned. It remains however a common means of dealing with the distress caused by anxiety disorders. Bolton et al.'s (2006) study examined the prevalence of self-medicating anxiety through the use of alcohol and drugs. People with generalized anxiety disorder had the highest prevalence of self-medication at 35.6% with *any* other anxiety disorder at 21.9%. Of particular concern was the finding that self-medicating behaviour remained significantly associated with an increased likelihood of suicidal ideation. An example of this can be seen with the 'Healthy Place' (2014) blog with a posting which outlines the difficulty of altering self-medicating behaviour once started, in this instance being caught in a downward spiral resulting in suicidal depression.

Members of the discussion forum on the Sober Recovery (2011) website reflect the issue that using alcohol to self-medicate for the effects of anxiety can provide temporary relief although it ultimately makes symptoms worse. A particular difficulty is the point of stopping drinking, a time which members highlighted as where their feelings of distress felt more severe. The issue being illustrated here is the desperate need to take control and gain relief from what can be torturous and truly distressing symptoms. Having achieved momentary respite it is indeed very hard to contemplate sobriety with all of one's worries and negative feelings emerging. Members also shared how immersed they could become in regrets of the past and worries for the future. However, not drinking enabled some members to discover more productive coping mechanisms such as relaxation and breathing exercises. It is a very hard cycle to break out of for those with anxiety disorders as self-medicating through using alcohol or drugs can increase a person's risk of developing incident substance use disorders (Robinson et al., 2009a). Robinson et al. (2009b) examined the prevalence and co-morbidity of self-medication for anxiety disorders. Rates of self-medication with alcohol were highest for those with GAD (18.5%) and social phobia (16.9%). Highest rates for self-medication with drugs (with or without the use of alcohol additionally) were social phobia (4.5%) and GAD (5.1%).

Further discussion is provided by members of the Anxiety Central (2012) discussion forum:

> To ease my nerves and to help me be able to interact with others, I have a drink or two.
>
> I stopped drinking when my anxiety was at its worst. I found (drinking) made me more anxious. I'd get worried, paranoid and concerned about the feelings of losing control.

One member recounts drinking before attending lectures and smoking 'weed' in order to cope in public. It had a negative effect of being rude to people which subsequently impacted upon feelings:

> I will trade panic in a public setting to that any time.

This is evidently an insidious cycle which individuals can become trapped within, struggling to cope with problems caused by their anxiety as well as substances they are consuming in order to manage symptoms. The Anxiety and Depression Association of America (ADAA) indicate that for most people with alcohol or substance abuse and an anxiety disorder the symptoms of one disorder can make the symptoms of the other worse. Effective support would recognise the needs for temporary relief from distressing anxiety symptoms whilst at the same time working towards more sustainable outcomes.

SECTION 2: EXPERIENCING SUPPORT

Interview narratives

I had to do things [in CBT] that I didn't want to do, like challenging myself ... that requires a lot of effort and sometimes it's easier just to carry on in the familiar pattern of thinking.

I've tried group therapy ... they crammed a lot of us into a little room and people had to walk out and leave because they were too anxious. It needed to be one on one.

I always got the impression when I got to see psychiatrists that they'd already made their mind up before I sat down and I always got the impression that they weren't listening really.

A major thing was joining a therapeutic community and being with other people who were suffering to an equal degree which allowed me to get a bit of perspective on what I was going through.

I've tried talking therapies and incidentally it was with psychoanalysis that I had someone I felt I had a real connection with.

In one particular therapy session we went off script and there was a genuineness there ... we joked about a Judas Priest song called 'Breaking the Law' and it felt like in that moment, we had much more of a perspective on things.

You name it I've been on it ... my experience of medication is that they hope it's a magic bullet and it's cheaper than offering you counselling.

I am currently on medication which I find helpful for taking the edge off things without feeling too vague or zoned out.

A bit of me felt like taking medication would make me a failure, like why can't I control this myself. It's that negative self-doubt and critical thinking.

I read other people's stories on a website panic.com where we all sit and terrify each other.

> *Through doing volunteering I have met a whole new group of people … they're obviously experiencing similar things themselves so they can understand and can be quite supportive when you are going through a difficult time.*
>
> *Art has been important.*

The main treatment options offered to those experiencing anxiety disorders include psychological therapies (cognitive behavioural therapy [CBT], exposure and response prevention therapy [ERP], psycho-education, applied relaxation, debriefing and trauma-focused work) and medication (antidepressants, beta blockers and tranquillisers) (NICE, 2011). Treatment choices are commonly CBT/ERP or medication or a combination of both. There have been a number of studies comparing the efficacy of CBT against medication with mixed results. Beidel et al. (2007) compared selective serotonin reuptake inhibitors (SSRIs) to CBT in the treatment of SAD in children and adolescents and found CBT to be more effective at the end of the treatment phase. Walkup et al. (2009) however found no difference in outcome between those treated with Sertraline and those treated with CBT. Cuijpers et al. (2013) found that the differences in effects between psychotherapy and antidepressant medication were small to non-existent for panic disorder and SAD and that psychotherapy was significantly more efficacious in OCD. The narratives from those on the receiving end from various treatments are outlined in the following text and expand this evaluation further. This is complemented by a discussion of other important interventions such as the support obtained through creative interventions (i.e. art and music) or through involvement with peers/individuals with shared experience of anxiety problems. Hospitalisation, a less common intervention than medication or psychotherapy is experienced by some when problems are sufficiently severe and individuals are unable to cope.

PSYCHOLOGICAL THERAPIES

What help would you want if seeking support from psychological/talking therapies?

Alongside pharmaceutical interventions, psychological talking therapies offer key treatment support for anxiety disorders. There are a variety of different psychotherapeutic interventions utilised which include low intensity (guided self-help, exposure therapy, problem solving, sleep hygiene and cognitive restructuring) and high intensity (mindfulness and acceptance based interventions) interventions (Askey-Jones and Askey-Jones, 2013). These are offered alongside other interventions such as ERP, psycho-education, applied relaxation, debriefing and trauma-focused work. Recovery rates empirically support the use of psychological treatments for anxiety (Richards and Borglin, 2011). Whilst NICE (2014) strongly advocates the use of psychotherapeutic interventions with anxiety disorders, there are a number of obstacles with their uptake. Creswell et al. (2014) found a large number of young people with anxiety disorders not accessing support due to a lack of awareness of knowledge and services, long waiting lists, competing family time commitments and a paucity of trained professionals. Another issue to consider concerns those dropping out of therapy, which according to Taylor et al. (2012) include low treatment motivation and practical barriers to attending sessions.

The process of therapy can be arduous and emotionally challenging although beneficial if worked through. One blogger found her therapy at times very hard as well as upsetting although ultimately transformative. She feels that the support gained through the therapeutic process was instrumental in developing a series of helpful coping strategies (Time to Change, 2014c). Kant (2008) expresses the value for him from psychotherapy which helped to reduce the potency of his obsessional thoughts as well as learning how to tune them out. These narratives illustrate some important psychotherapeutic goals relating to the development of personal mastery over troubling thoughts as well as reducing the impact from troubling anxiety symptoms.

The discussion threads on the SAUK website illustrate some interesting responses to psychological care. For a number of people, opening up about one's problems and sharing them with a therapist was regarded as liberating. This included aspects which individuals had been struggling with alone for some time. The point of finally receiving support felt a relief and was greatly welcomed. Other postings though highlighted difficulties with not feeling supported or safe with their therapists. Interestingly, some found it easier and more beneficial sharing experiences on the discussion forum with fellow members, people who they could relate to and whom they felt understood by. When understanding and connectedness are encountered through the psychotherapeutic process the response can be very appreciative:

> The first few sessions were a revelation; to be able to talk freely to someone who really understood what I was going through, who didn't seem to think I was crazy and who reassured me that not only was OCD way more common than I'd ever thought, but more importantly that there was a way of beating it and changing for the better.
>
> Veale and Willson (2011, p. 34)

This strongly illustrates feelings of hope which have been created through the shared interpersonal work being done. The therapist's approach and personal qualities are also important in terms of an individual's continued engagement. Daisy Fields (2002) encountered numerous psychotherapeutic approaches including Freudian psychoanalysis, behavioural therapy and cognitive therapy. All of these were regarded as useful although what stood out the most for her was the warm, accepting manner of one of her therapists, something she regarded as very helpful in fostering her self-esteem. The OCD Action (2015) online discussion forum illustrates some interesting views about therapy. Learning how to relax, coping with anxiety symptoms and feeling heard were generally acknowledged as effective outcomes. A range of difficulties though were encountered in connection with the organisational process with particular emphasis placed upon waiting times. This was illustrated through a number of concerns over having waited months for an assessment and then a further few months before the start of treatment.

It can potentially encourage attrition and 'no shows' coupled with the feelings of apprehension and uncertainty felt at the start of therapy:

> I'm gonna be doing some stuff to make me anxious in the coming weeks, and
> I feel very, very scared.

Clearly, therapists need to be mindful of these fears as well what is experienced through therapeutic work. The discomfort felt needs to be managed carefully so as to allow for engagement with the therapeutic activities to develop. As Muir-Cochrane (2009) highlights, people with anxiety problems may initially find it difficult to complete suggested tasks and to practice relaxation methods they have been encouraged to use. This is a key issue, considering how frustrated, disheartened or useless individuals can feel if therapy does not seem to be working. The point though at which progress is noted can be uplifting and motivational. Rose Bretécher (2013) found ERP to be life-changing and inspiring of hope as it enabled her to reach a position of tolerance with her feelings of anxiety instead of engaging her compulsions:

> Slowly I found myself less and less anxious in response to the stimuli. Just letting the thoughts 'be there' without questioning them was the essential skill which would help me manage my condition in future.

This illustrates the process of understanding which ERP applies to the OCD cycle, thereby enabling personal change (Olson et al., 2007). It reflects elements contained within other psychotherapeutic approaches which facilitate insight gaining, mastery and control over anxiety as well as relief and respite from troubling symptoms. Other important aspects include then sense of acceptance and understanding attained through being 'heard' by someone they do not feel critically judged by. This enables individuals to feel safe and hopeful which helps them cope with the difficulty and emotional stress of therapy and work towards achieving effective change. A final narrative concerning the benefits of psychotherapy can be given to Emily Ford who relates:

> With proper treatment, it's possible to have a rich, rewarding, socially active life. My anxiety is unlikely to disappear completely, especially in times of stress. But now I'm prepared with strategies for handling it and I know where to turn if help is required.
>
> Ford et al. (2007, p. 9)

MEDICATION

Medication prescribed to people experiencing anxiety disorders involves different types which are indicated by NICE (2014) as follows:

Antidepressants: SSRIs are mainly used to treat depression although they are also used with various anxiety disorders. They work by increasing the levels of serotonin, a neurotransmitter which influences mood, emotion and sleep.

Beta blockers: Physical symptoms of anxiety such as rapid heartbeat, palpitations and tremor can be treated with beta blockers. Their success is variable and they do not reduce the psychological symptoms of anxiety.

Tranquillisers and sleeping pills: These offer temporary measure for severe or disabling anxiety. Withdrawal symptoms though can feel worse than the original feelings of anxiety. Long-term use of tranquillisers has been linked with panic attacks.

A study conducted by Wilson et al. (2014) showed evidence of significant anxiety symptom reduction from short-term medication use. Their effectiveness can also be gauged through personal narratives, acknowledging the impact that this treatment modality has upon individuals' day-to-day functioning. Experiences on the whole show a broad range of experience with mixed views about the impact upon their lives. Discussion threads on the SAUK (2014) website reveal both positive and negative experiences. The medication types and dosages prescribed varied significantly illustrating clearly the different needs and responses to mediation types. There was some commonality expressed with regards to the function that medication had in terms of 'taking the edge' off one's anxiety and reducing the feelings of timidity, uncertainty and tension experienced in a range of situations. Particular problems and concerns related to side effects with tiredness, feeling mentally sluggish or 'zombified' echoed through a number of postings. This was met with discussion around alternative treatment and remedies with a number of individuals contemplating reducing dosages or stopping altogether. Problems with side effects influenced non-compliance with medication as illustrated in a study by Taylor et al. (2012). It is perhaps useful to consider some of the associated side effects connected with anti-anxiolytic medication. Common side effects, for example, with benzodiazepines or tranquilisers include the following:

- Drowsiness, lack of energy
- Clumsiness, slow reflexes
- Slurred speech
- Confusion and disorientation
- Depression
- Dizziness, light-headedness
- Impaired thinking and judgment
- Memory loss, forgetfulness
- Nausea, stomach upset
- Blurred or double vision (Help Guide, 2015)

How would you feel about taking medication if faced with this list?

Other identified problems with medication used to treat anxiety include their addictive nature and dependency problems linked with pharmacological agents such as benzodiazepines have made clinicians reluctant to prescribe them (Von Moltke and Greenblatt, 2003). Withdrawal from other medication types can also cause difficulties as discussion threads on the Patient discussion forum reveal. One particular discussion around withdrawal from Citalopram (SSRI antidepressant) shows experiences with severe mood swings, suicidal thoughts, dizziness, nausea, tearfulness, irritability, anger, and head-aches. There was also for some a demoralising return of anxiety symptoms. This can be contrasted against the relief experienced in feeling less 'fuzzy', having renewed appetite for life and significantly the ability to cry again:

> I don't want to go back on the pills, it is lovely to cry again at a film.

The available narratives highlight a wide range of experiences either through taking medication, reducing dosages or stopping altogether. They also highlight the need for more information about the effects and what can be expected from taking different types of medication. Information is shared freely within peer support networks such as discussion forums and whilst including a lot of helpful support a certain amount of misinformation is also circulated. What is lacking is sustained clarification around medication effects from health care professionals, something a number of people are not receiving. Wells (2006, p. 83) describes being insufficiently informed about the medication offered by his doctor:

> My fears were that either I would feel artificially 'happy' and would walk around wearing a big false smile or that my feelings would be deadened and I wouldn't feel like myself anymore.

Therefore, it is vital that practitioners not only give detailed information but also check service users' understanding and provide space for questions and expression of fears.

IN-PATIENT CARE

Hospital admissions for anxiety are found to increase with age being highest among older women. The most common age group for male admissions to hospital was 45–49 years (Health and Social Care Information Centre, 2014). A question posed on the Anxiety Zone discussion forum asks peers whether anyone has been hospitalised through problems with anxiety. The responses reveal various numbers of visits to the ER department but only brief admissions to hospital. There are a number of discussion threads noted with members speculating about what hospital admission would involve with a number of stereotypical thoughts shared. Some of these postings reveal a significant level of concern about in-patient care although in most instances information is based upon second-hand reports. In terms of the reality of hospital care we can consider the service offered by the UK's Bethlem Royal Hospital which has a specialist unit for treating people experiencing anxiety problems. Jo (National Services, 2015) provides a narrative account of her satisfaction with the service provided stating how important it was to feel connected and understood by others. She also highlighted the value in feeling secure, supported and having people to talk with whenever needed. A discussion thread around hospital care on the Healing Well (2009) discussion forum details inclusion within a wide variety of individual and group activities such as yoga, meditation and exercise. Particular mention was made of group psychotherapy where personal experiences with anxiety were shared and discussed. The feelings around one's admission to hospital illustrated contrasting experiences:

It really made me worse at first with fear, although after two weeks, I ended up afraid to leave and go back in the real world.

It was nothing like 'one flew over the cuckoos nest'. It was helpful, encouraging and great to meet others who shared the same fears. No-one judged anyone. That's my experience, and I feel blessed that I found a place that can treat me without making me feel like a freak.

These narratives show how diversely different people's experience of hospital care can be. If effectively delivered, this time can provide much needed respite and acknowledgement of one's difficulties. Feeling accepted and 'normal' is important to people who have perhaps experienced a fair degree of stigmatisating and dismissive treatment from others. Hospital care can therefore offer a refuge when feeling overwhelmed and in need of more intense support or can exacerbate feelings of unease and distress.

CREATIVE EXPRESSION

Further therapeutic opportunities are embraced through a range of creative outlets such as music, art, dance, poetry and literature. This provides people with a means of expression as well as engagement with creative modes which have a relaxing or distracting effect. Artwork, for example, can work well here through the process of construction or the impact that various pieces have upon a person's environment. A study by Nanda et al. (2011) concluded that positive distractions from visual art can help to reduce levels of anxiety and agitation in healthcare settings. McKella Sawyer (2015) writes:

I've found that the best way to calm that anxious mind is to actually be creative and make stuff ... Sometimes all you need to do is let that fear out where you can see it, onto a canvas or a blank page, where it's easier to deal with than when it's lurking in the back of your mind.

A notable event providing breadth of artistic expression was the Anxiety Arts Festival (Mental Health Foundation, 2014) held in London exploring anxiety as a modern condition. This incorporated a range of visual and performance arts activities along with film screenings and creative writing workshops.

Music is another creative mode which can have strong therapeutic benefits. Becky (Your Stories, 2014a) expresses the importance of music for her:

Music has been a vital conduit for self-expression, relaxation and comfort ... Song-writing ended up being a healthy outlet for me to express myself and helped me to understand the way I think and deal with things... music has helped me get through some of my darkest times.

Music provides an avenue for expression and a means of coping with difficult and distressing emotions. Indeed, Choi et al.'s (2008) study involving a music intervention group showed significant improvements in depression and anxiety. Another study by Gutiérrez and Camarena (2015) found music therapy to be an effective means of reducing anxiety and depression levels in GAD patients.

There are a number of poems about the experience of anxiety on the website Family Friend Poems. They include some very expressive accounts such as Mysterious Pain, The Mysterious Pain, The Girl I Used to Be PTSD or Panic Disorder. This evidently provides an important outlet for expression which is rich in symbolic imagery. It also provides others with a means of engaging with a person's internal experience of anxiety. The importance of such means of expression is being increasingly recognised for their educational and health promotional value. Events such as the annual Love Arts Festival, held in Leeds promote thinking about mental health experience, including problems with anxiety, through the use of the arts. They offer a range of expressive modes such as drama, art, music, film, photography, literature, poetry and dance. It is clear that more creative interventions are needed both as a means for helping those with anxiety problems as well as others in terms of enhancing understanding and reducing stigma.

PEER SUPPORT

> What benefits do you feel individuals with anxiety can get through contact with peers (others experiencing problems with anxiety)?

As with other mental health problems, there are a growing number of initiatives and resources offering opportunities for peer support for those with anxiety disorders. This is where help is sought (and given) in relation to other individuals who have shared experience of problems with anxiety. The range of support and resources available include face-to-face self-help groups, family and friends as well as a steadily growing number of online resources. Online discussion forums such as SAUK, OCD Action and Anxiety Central provide important space for members to share information, ask questions and receive help. These environments provide opportunities for people to feel acknowledged, understood and connected with others. This fosters a sense of universality, the feeling that one is not alone (Yalom, 2005). The SAUK chatroom illustrates the widespread use of this resource with thousands of posts and discussion threads available. The value to members of this resource is shown in the following posting:

> This website is great, it is nice to have somewhere to be able to chat to people who know exactly what it feels like and the problems faced, as there is nobody else who would understand.

Also the feeling of engagement with other people is the acknowledgement that others understand what one is experiencing. A clear function of these discussion forums is the reciprocal nature of both supporting others and being supported by them. Offering help enables people to feel valued and appreciated which in turn will impact upon self-esteem. It is also notable that the support which one can offer seems to be an important point in a person's recovery. This becomes empowering and morale boosting and can be realised through a variety of initiatives either online or within one's local community. Stephen (Your Stories, 2014b) recounts:

> One of the biggest things that has helped to bring me out of myself and build confidence is all the volunteering work I do.

This included co-presenting a radio show for local radio and involvement with mental health advocacy groups Time to Change and Young Minds. Other narratives illustrate how engaging with others through a reciprocal relationship can be enormously beneficial. Claire (NHS Choices, 2014b) was diagnosed with agoraphobia after experiencing a panic attack while shopping. She gradually stopped going out only truly feeling safe at home dependent on elderly neighbours to buy food and household supplies. CBT was not particularly effective for her, and what made the difference was sharing her experience with others experiencing anxiety problems whom she contacted through support groups on the Internet:

> You feel like a freak ... Talking to other people in the same position was what helped me most.

This led to a reciprocal arrangement with another person experiencing similar problems to her. They supported each other making similar steps in their respective neighbourhoods, encouraging each other to slowly increase the time and length of their journeys. This, along with other narrative accounts, points towards important aspects in a person's recovery. It concerns the sense of connection that is established with others who understand what one is going through as well as feeling productive and valued. This enables one to take control over their difficulties and is a big change from the feelings of helplessness and impotence which are central to many anxiety disorders. It is imperative therefore that healthcare professionals recognise this need and facilitate opportunities for individuals to take personal control within one's own care as well as having opportunities to productively assist others in whatever capacity seems most appropriate.

SECTION 3: LIVING WELL

Interview narratives

I have a network of people who have been with me in the therapeutic community and I can speak to them on bad days.

Relationships where people can help each other are vital.

I think for me what is important is having a sense of belonging and feeling accepted.

I'm trying to accept and accept myself for who I am. I'm trying to come to terms that there are always going to be things that might be restricted ... but it doesn't mean that I won't achieve things or have a normal kind of life.

Recovery from anxiety problems will mean different things to different people. The emphasis here though is on well-being and achieving the best possible level of functioning. Whilst in some cases this might involve feeling free of distressing symptoms for others it might involve learning how to live with difficulties and find ways of re-engaging in one's life. Living well can also relate to reaching a position of acceptance:

> I used to long for the day I'd be cured … But part of my recovery was accepting how unrealistic this was, and I'm now completely at peace with the idea that I'll probably always have OCD to some extent.

> Bretécher (2013)

Another key aspect concerns personal gains achieved through the process of working through one's difficulties and developing new adaptive coping methods. A service user in Veale and Willson's (2011, p. 81) text, whilst expressing the ravages that anxiety problems have visited upon his life, also reflects upon their 'silver lining' and the opportunities to develop

> vast amounts of wisdom, knowledge and a perspective that allows me to look at life with an open mind.

Likewise, Peter (OCD Action, 2015) states:

> I hate to say it, but OCD has taught me a lot too. It's helped me to see that almost everything has positives and despite any overwhelming negatives they need to be retained if there is to be any benefit.

These narratives view the anxiety experience as a potential catalyst for learning and change. This is illustrated by Peterson (2015) in her 'Anxiety-Schmanxiety' blog who details the various things she has learnt which concern her mind, body and whole being. These illustrate new ways of framing and conceptualising her thoughts, feelings and physical sensations. They also communicate resilience, thoughtfulness and optimism for the future. This conveys a sense of hope that problems can be challenged and that there is a potential to live well with anxiety. This is shared through a number of narratives recounting daily experiences in recovery. In his blog, 'Doug' (I Am Living With Anxiety, 2015) shares a number of accounts concerned with his handling of distressing thoughts, coping with anxiety-provoking experiences and recognising and dealing with bodily symptoms. It is an expressive and accessible blog providing a sense of hope and the belief that constructive, purposeful and enjoyable lives can be lived, even if challenged with anxiety provoking symptoms. There is an indication here of the greater feelings of self-control that can be attained along with the creation of adaptive coping skills. Ellen's (2015) experience of the gains through psychotherapy is illustrative of this, developing skills to manage stressful situations over and above those connected with her anxiety problems.

Living well significantly involves engagement and contact with others. Having people whom individuals can express themselves openly to and feel accepted by helps to 'normalise' experience and as related through a number of narratives enable them to feel less 'freakish'. Reciprocal support as achieved with peers is highly important and instrumental in maintaining well-being and developing confidence and self-esteem. A core element concerns the feeling of productivity through being able to offer support to others. This significantly lowers dependency and helplessness which is commonly experienced with anxiety. There is also the added bonus of feeling needed, appreciated and valued by others. These elements are all part of sustainable and adaptive coping methods which work. They can be combined with a reduction in feelings of helplessness and developing feelings of self-control. It all combines to enable a person to have an enhanced sense of resilience and hope showing that with appropriate support individuals can attain a position of acceptance and means of fulfilling personal potential.

How do you feel about the narratives expressed in this section?

REFERENCES

ADAA (2014a). Achieving happiness. http://www.adaa.org, accessed 17 February, 2015.

ADAA (2014b). My journey to peace. http://www.adaa.org, accessed 17 February, 2015.

ADAA (2014c). The 4-word message on a ribbon that helps me with anxiety. http://www.adaa.org, accessed 17 February, 2015.

ADAA (2014d). My story of survival: Battling PTSD. http://www.adaa.org, accessed 17 February, 2015.

ADAA. (2015). Anxiety disorder or substance abuse: Which comes first? http://www.adaa.org, accessed 20 July, 2015.

American Psychiatric Association (2013). DSM-5. http://www.dsm5.org, accessed 16 April, 2015.

Anxiety Central (2012). Using alcohol to self-medicate. http://www.anxiety-central.com, accessed 27 August, 2015.

Anxiety Forum. (2015). Forum. http://anxietyforum.net/forum/forum.php, accessed 29 May, 2015.

Anxiety Zone. (2015). Forum. http://www.anxietyzone.com, accessed 22 July, 2015.

Askey-Jones, S. and Askey-Jones, R. (2013). The person with an anxiety disorder. In I. Norman and I. Ryrie (Eds.), *The Art and Science of Mental Health Nursing* (3rd ed., pp. 569–586). Open University Press: Maidenhead, England.

Beidel, D., Turner, S., Sallee, F.R., Ammerman, R.T., Crosby, L.A. and Pathak, S. (2007). SET-C versus fluoxetine in the treatment of childhood social phobia. *Journal of the American Academy of Child & Adolescent Psychiatry.* 46, 1622–1632.

Bolton, J., Cox, B., Clara, I. and Sareen, J. (2006). Use of alcohol and drugs to self-medicate anxiety disorders in a nationally representative Sample. *The Journal of Nervous and Mental Disease.* 194(11), 818–825.

Bourne, E. (2011). *The Anxiety and Phobia Workbook* (5th ed). New Harbinger Publications: Oakland, CA.

Bretécher, R. (2013). Pure OCD. A rude awakening http://www.theguardian.com, accessed 11 July, 2014.

Buchanan, H. and Coulson, N. (2012). *Phobias.* Palgrave Macmillan: London, UK.

Choi, A., Lee, M. and Lim, H. (2008). Effects of group music intervention on depression, anxiety, and relationships in psychiatric patients: A pilot study. *The Journal of Alternative and Complementary Medicine.* 14(5), 567–570.

Clerkin, E.M., Smith, A.R. and Hames, J.L. (2014). The interpersonal effects of Facebook reassurance seeking. *Journal of Affective Disorders.* 151(2), 525–530.

Corrigan, P.W., Larson, J.E. and Rüsch, N. (2009). Self-stigma and the "why try" effect: Impact on life goals and evidence-based practices. *World Psychiatry.* 8(2), 75–81.

Creswell, C., Waite, P. and Cooper, P. (2014). Assessment and management of anxiety disorders in children and adolescents. *Archives of Disease in Childhood*. 99, 674–678.

Cuijpers, P., Sijbrandij, M., Koole, S., Andersson, G., Beekman, A. and Reynolds, C. (2013). The efficacy of psychotherapy and pharmacotherapy in treating depressive and anxiety disorders: A meta-analysis of direct comparisons. *World Psychiatry*. 12(2), 137–148.

Daily Mail (2014). She must Brie terrified. http://www.dailymail.co.uk, accessed 27 August, 2015.

Ellen (2015). Will my OCD ever go away? https://ellensocdblog.wordpress.com, accessed 19 October, 2015.

Family Friend Poems. (2015). Loving, healing, touching. http://www.familyfriendpoems.com, accessed 21 August, 2015.

Fennell, D. and Liberato, A.S.Q. (2007). Learning to live with OCD: Labeling, the self, and stigma. *Deviant Behavior*. 28(4), 305–331.

Fields, D. (2002). Living with obsessive compulsive disorder. In R. Ramsay, A. Page, T. Goodman and D. Hart (Eds.), *Changing Minds* (pp. 47–50). Gaskell: London, UK.

Ford, E., Liebowitz, M. and Andrews, W. (2007). *What You Must Think of Me*. Oxford University Press: Oxford, UK.

Gale, C. and Davidson, O. (2007). Generalised anxiety disorder. *British Medical Journal*. 334, 579.

Gekoski, A. and Broome, S. (2014). *What's Normal Anyway. Celebrities Own Stories of Mental Illness*. Constable: London, UK.

Gutiérrez, E.O. and Camarena, V.A. (2015). Music therapy in generalized anxiety disorder. *The Arts in Psychotherapy*. 15, 19–24.

Hapke, U., Schumann, A., Rumpf, H., John, U. and Meyer, C. (2006). Post-traumatic stress disorder. *European Archive of Psychiatry and Clinical Neuroscience*. 256, 99–306.

Healing Well (2009). Hospitalisation for anxiety... What will happen to me? http://www.healingwell.com, accessed 16 April, 2015.

Health and Social Care Information Centre (2014). Anxiety: Hospital admissions highest in women in their late 60s. http://www.hscic.gov.uk, accessed 16 April, 2015.

Healthy Place (2014). What happens when an addict self-medicates for anxiety? http://www.healthyplace.com, accessed 27 August, 2015.

Help Guide (2015). Anxiety medication. http://www.helpguide.org, accessed 15 December, 2015.

I Am Living With Anxiety (2015). I am living with anxiety. http://iamlivingwithanxiety.blogspot.co.uk, accessed 14 September, 2015.

Isensee, B., Wittchen, H., Stein, M.B., Höfler, M. and Lieb, R. (2003). Smoking increases the risk of panic. Findings from a prospective community study. *Archives of General Psychiatry*. 60(7), 692–700.

Kant, J. (2008). *The Thought that Counts: A Firsthand Account of One Teenager's Experience with Obsessive-Compulsive Disorder*. Oxford University Press: Oxford, UK.

Kaye, W.H., Bulik, C.M., Thornton, L., Barbarich, N. and Masters, K. (2004). Comorbidity of anxiety disorders with anorexia and bulimia nervosa. *The American Journal of Psychiatry*. 161(12), 2215–2221.

Kendall, T., Cape, J., Chan, M. and Taylor, C. (2011). Management of generalised anxiety disorder in adults: Summary of NICE guidance. *British Medical Journal*. 342, c7460.

King, D.B. and Wertheimer, M. (2007). *Max Wertheimer and Gestalt Theory*. Transaction Publishers: New Brunswick, NJ.

Love Arts. (2015). http://loveartsleeds.co.uk, accessed 3 November, 2015.

Masellis, M., Rector, N.A. and Richter, M.A. (2003). Quality of life in OCD: Differential impact of obsessions, compulsions, and depression comorbidity. *Canadian Journal of Psychiatry*. 48(2), 72–77.

McLean, D. (2014). *Overcoming Panic Disorder. My Story–My Journey. Into and beyond Anxiety, Panic Attacks and Agoraphobia*. Balboa: Bloomington, IN.

Mental Health Foundation (2014). Anxiety Arts Festival. http://www.anxietyartsfestival.org, accessed 16 April, 2015.

Millwallant (2013). OCD Awareness Week. http://www.ocduk, accessed 11 July, 2014.

Mind (2013a). Anxiety. http://www.mind.org.uk, accessed 17 November, 2014.

Mind (2013b). Internal conflict of an anxious mind. http://www.mind.org.uk, accessed 1 March, 2014.

Mind (2013c). Sleeping with anxiety. http://www.mind.org, accessed 1 March, 2014.

Mind (2014). Managing anxiety with creativity. http://www.mind.org, accessed 30 October, 2015.

Muir-Cochrane, E. (2009). The person who experiences anxiety. In P. Barker (Ed.), *Psychiatric and Mental Health Nursing* (2nd ed., pp. 165–172). Hodder Arnold: London, UK.

Nanda, U., Eisen, S., Zadeh, R. and Owen, D. (2011). Effect of visual art on patient anxiety and agitation in a mental health facility and implications for the business case. *Journal of Psychiatric and Mental Health Nursing*. 18(5), 386–393.

National Institute of Mental Health (2015). General; Anxiety disorder. http://www.nimh.nih.gov, accessed 8 September, 2015.

National Services (2015). Jo's Story. http://www.national.slam.nhs.uk, accessed 16 April, 2015.

NHS Choices (2013). Post-traumatic stress disorder (PTSD). http://www.nhs.uk, accessed 16 April, 2015.

NHS Choices (2014a). Generalised anxiety disorder in adults. http://www.nhs.uk, accessed 16 April, 2015.

NHS Choices (2014b). I beat agoraphobia. www.nhs.uk, accessed 16 April, 2015.

NICE (2011). Generalized anxiety disorder and panic disorder. https://www.nice.org.uk, accessed 16 April, 2015.

NICE (2013). Social anxiety disorder: Recognition, assessment and treatment. https://www.nice.org.uk, accessed 16 April, 2015.

NICE (2014). New NICE quality standard aims to improve recognition, assessment and availability of treatments for anxiety disorders. https://www.nice.org.uk, accessed 16 April, 2015.

O'Brien, C. (2011). Anxiety was my prison. http://www.dailymail.co.uk, accessed 7 June, 2014.

OCD Action (2008). Forum. http://www.ocdaction.org.uk, accessed 12 September, 2015.

OCD Action (2015). Forum. http://www.ocdaction.org.uk, accessed 12 September, 2015.

OCDLA (2010). Reassurance seeking in OCD and anxiety. http://ocdla.com, accessed 16 April, 2015.

OCD UK (2014). So OCD, is it a laughing matter? http://www.ocduk, accessed 16 April, 2015.

Olson, T., Vera, B. and Perez, O. (2007). From primetime to paradise; the lived experience of OCD in Hawaii. *Family & Community Health*. 30(2), 59–70.

Peterson, T. (2015). Lessons I've learned from anxiety. http://www.healthyplace.com, accessed 26 September, 2015.

Phobia Fear Release (2014). Fear of pigeons. http://www.phobia-fear-release.com, accessed 3 April, 2015.

Richards, D. and Borglin, G. (2011). Implementation of psychological therapies for anxiety and depression in routine practice: Two year prospective cohort study. *Journal of Affective Disorders*. 133(1–2), 51–60.

Robinson, J., Sareen, J., Cox, B. and Bolton, J. (2009a). Correlates of self-medication for anxiety disorders: Results from the national epidemiologic survey on alcohol and related conditions. *The Journal of Nervous and Mental Disease*. 197, 873–878.

Robinson, J., Sareen, J., Cox, B. and Bolton, J. (2009b). Self-medication of anxiety disorders with alcohol and drugs: Results from a nationally representative sample. *Journal of Anxiety Disorders*. 23(1), 38–45.

SAUK (2014). Discussion board. http://www.social-anxiety.org.uk, accessed 12 September, 2015.

Sawyer, M. (2015). How art can heal anxiety. http://www.thechangeblog.com, accessed 26 September, 2015.

Sober Recovery (2011). Alcohol self-medication. http://www.soberrecovery.com, accessed 16 April, 2015.

Stein, M., Roy-Byrne, P., Craske, M., Campbell-Sills, L., Lang, A., Golinelli, D. et al. (2012). Quality of and patient satisfaction with primary health care for anxiety disorders. *Journal of Clinical Psychiatry*. 72(7), 970–976.

Stein, M. and Stein, D.J. (2008). Social anxiety disorder. *The Lancet*. 371(9618), 1115–1125.

Swinbourne, J.M. and Touyz, S.W. 2007. The comorbidity of eating disorders and anxiety disorders: A review. *European Eating Disorders Review*. 15(4), 253–274.

Taylor, S., Abramowitz, J. and McKay, D. (2012). Non-adherence and non-response in the treatment of anxiety disorders. *Journal of Anxiety Disorders*. 26(5), 583–589.

Time to Change (2012a). Personal narrative. http://www.time-to-change.org.uk, accessed 22 April, 2015.

Time to Change (2012b). Personal narrative. http://www.time-to-change.org.uk, accessed 22 April, 2015.

Time to Change (2013a). Personal narrative. http://www.time-to-change.org.uk, accessed 25 April, 2015.

Time to Change (2013b). Personal narrative. http://www.time-to-change.org.uk, accessed 25 April, 2015.

Time to Change (2013c). Personal narrative. http://www.time-to-change.org.uk, accessed 25 April, 2015.

Time to Change (2013d). Personal narrative. http://www.time-to-change.org.uk, accessed 25 April, 2015.

Time to Change (2013e). Personal narrative. http://www.time-to-change.org.uk, accessed 25 April, 2015.

Time to Change (2014a). Personal narrative. http://www.time-to-change.org.uk, accessed 16 April, 2015.

Time to Change (2014b). Personal narrative. http://www.time-to-change.org, accessed 16 April, 2015.

Time to Change (2014c). Personal narrative. http://www.time-to-change.org, accessed 16 April, 2015.

Time to Change (2014d). Personal narrative. http://www.time-to-change.org, accessed 16 April, 2015.

Turk, C., Heimberg, R. and Magee, L. (2008). Social anxiety disorder. In D. Barlow (Ed.), *Clinical Handbook of Psychological Disorders* (4th ed., pp. 123–163). The Guilford Press: New York.

Tyrer, P. and Baldwin, D. (2006). Generalised anxiety disorder. *The Lancet* 368(9553), 2156–2166.

Veale, D. and Willson, R. (Eds.). (2011). *Taking Control of OCD: Inspirational Stories of Hope and Recovery*. Robinson: London, UK.

Von Moltke, L. and Greenblatt, D. (2003). Medication dependence and anxiety. *Dialogues in Clinical Neuroscience*. 5(3), 237–245.

Walkup, J., Albano, A., Piacentini, J., Birmaher, B., Compton, S.N., Sherriff, J.T. et al. (2009). Cognitive behavioural therapy, Sertraline, or a combination in childhood anxiety. *New England Journal of Medicine*. 359, 2753–2766.

Waters, A. and Craske, M. (2005). Generalised anxiety disorder. In M. Anthony, D. Ledley and R. Heimberg (Eds.), *Improving Outcomes and Preventing Relapse in Cognitive Behavioural Therapy* (pp. 77–126). Guilford Press: London, UK.

Wells, J. (2006). *Touch and Go Joe*. Jessica Kingsley Publishers: London, UK.

Wilson, H., Mannix, S., Oko-osi, H. and Revicki, D. (2014). The impact of medication on health-related quality of life in patients with generalized anxiety disorder. *CNS Drugs*. 29, 29–40.

Yalom, I. (2005). *Theory and Practice of Group Psychotherapy* (5th ed.). Basic Books: New York.

Your Stories (2012a). Simon Buckden. http://www.leedsandyorkpft.nhs.uk, accessed 16 April, 2015.

Your Stories (2012b). Rich Hilson. http://www.leedsandyorkpft.nhs.uk, accessed 16 April, 2015.

Your Stories (2014a). Becky Holt. http://www.leedsandyorkpft.nhs.uk, accessed 16 April, 2015.

Your Stories (2014b). Stephen Cross. http://www.leedsandyorkpft.nhs.uk, accessed 16 April, 2015.

'Walking in treacle'
Living with depression

INTRODUCTION

This chapter focuses upon the personal experience of individuals who are struggling to cope when mood states become depressed. It explores this from a *lived* and *felt* context and what having depression means to different people. The three sections within the chapter will cover the lived experience of depression, the experience of diagnosis and care and the conceptual meaning of one's total experience including recovery. Manifestations of depressive mood states are manifold, and likewise the causes of depression are hugely variable. Whilst addressing a significant range of issues, it is not possible within the space available in this chapter to cover all manifestations or experiences connected with depression. In addition, there is also substantial overlap with other health states and aspects such as psychotic experience and anxiety which are covered in greater depth in other chapters.

> Write down what you know about depression.
>
> What do you envisage the lived and felt experience entailing?

WHAT IS DEPRESSION?

Depression is one of the priority conditions covered by the World Health Authority's (WHO, 2014) Mental Health Gap Action Programme and is the top global cause of illness and disability for adolescents, with suicide the third biggest cause of death. It is a commonly experienced mental health problem with an estimated 350 million people affected worldwide (WHO, 2012). People from all demographic groups are affected (NAMI, 2015), and it is the second most common cause of disability after back pain (Ferrari et al., 2013). Approximately one-fifth of adults are affected by anxiety or depression (ONS, 2013), with around 80,000 children and young people suffering from severe depression (ONS, 2004). According to the World Health Authority (WHO, 2012) more women are affected by depression than men although this may be influenced by the greater tendency for women to disclose feelings and symptoms.

The term 'depression' is derived from the Latin word *deprimere* which means 'to press down' (Kanter et al., 2008). It is a common mental health problem characterised by sadness, loss of interest or pleasure, feelings of guilt or low self-worth, disturbed sleep or appetite, feelings of tiredness and poor concentration (Mind, 2012). Depression can last for weeks, months or years; it substantially impairs an individual's ability to cope with daily life and at its most severe can lead to suicide (Royal College of Psychiatrists, 2015a).

SECTION 1: EXPERIENCING DEPRESSION

Interview narratives

It got to the stage that I was missing deadlines, I knew I was stressed, I was weeping a lot … I was having nightmares about being found out that I was a fraud and not this super person.

All I wanted to do was curl up in bed and stay there.

I would describe it like walking in a sea of treacle. You don't want to get out of bed in the morning, everything is hard work … you don't want to move, you don't want to face the world, you don't want to speak to anybody, you just want to be isolated. It's awful.

Jobs that would have taken me half an hour to do took me half a day to do. Because you just can't concentrate on anything.

I wouldn't eat, not for a long time and lost a lot of weight. I just didn't want to eat.

The general public don't really understand that. They think if you're depressed you're having a bit of a bad day and they say snap out of it. But you can't.

I did attempt suicide … you can't see any way out of it, being in a big black hole and trying to crawl your way out if it but you can't. The more you try to crawl out the deeper you go into it. It's horrible.

When they [my friends] thought I were mentally ill they didn't want to know but when I had a stroke they all came around.

I started drinking very heavily … it made things worse although felt better at night because it would put me to sleep as I would be partly unconscious.

FIRST AWARENESS/INITIAL PROBLEMS

The first signs that one is suffering with depressive symptoms can be hard to identify given the myriad of potential causes which can be attributed to individual symptoms. Indeed, for William Styron (1990), depression was regarded as an elusive and mysterious condition with symptoms too subtle to initially notice. The changes taking place for him included a decline in energy levels, an increase in anxiety and a reduction in pleasure with previously enjoyed activities. Indeed the slow insidious progression of symptoms can explain why so many people struggle for years before contacting a professional (Brown et al., 2010). Rice-Oxley (2012) lists the impressions he had prior to his depressive 'breakdown' which included headaches, fatigue, surreal impressions of the world, restlessness, irritability, grumpiness, feelings of ambivalence, avoiding social situations and early wakening. Whilst collectively these symptoms can be viewed as problems with depression, taken individually they can be perfectly natural reactions to the everyday difficulties of life.

When considering health issues from a multidimensional, holistic perspective we can regard a number of elements such as physical, psychological, emotional, social and spiritual as interacting together (Landrum et al., 1993). The Royal College of Psychiatrists (2015a) indicate that a range of physical illnesses including cancer, heart disease, arthritis, viral infections and hormonal problems can cause depression. Interviewees on the Healthtalk online resource frequently reported physical ailments associated with their depression such as gastric upsets, back pain and fatigue. Whether physical problems lead to depressive feelings or vice versa will differ from person to person. A third of participants in Townend et al.'s (2010) study perceived themselves as 'useless' after a life event resulting in disability. Two-thirds of the participants however had a very different experience. A further issue to consider concerns the potential somatisation of emotional and psychological problems. The service user agency Beyond Blue (2015) lists physical symptoms as tiredness, nausea, headaches, muscle pains, sleep disturbance, changes in appetite, weight loss or gain. Physical ailments can feel less stigmatising and easier to accept, and Madhukar and Trivedi (2004) indicate that physical problems are commonly amongst the first presenting symptoms disclosed to healthcare professionals by people with depression. Ever since Freud developed his psychoanalytic theories through his work with patients like the infamous 'Dora', who suffered from amongst other things, migraines, loss of voice and fainting, inexplicable physical conditions have been linked to problems of the mind. A popular misconception is that the person realises they are doing this, are in control of the somatisation or are simply 'faking'. In fact, the somatisation of psychological states can act as a defensive mind–body split (Winnicott, 1964) which protects the person from unbearable states, albeit at a price. This defence may have its roots in previous trauma or could even be linked to the societal stigma surrounding psychological conditions. As Shapiro (2003, p. 549) succinctly states:

The shame must be addressed before the body and mind can be bridged.

When trying to make sense of causative factors, trauma, abuse, illness and disability can provide clear links with which to connect depressive feelings. Such experiences can have a major impact upon the person and severely disrupt their sense of equilibrium. Andrew Solomon (2002) relates his mother's diagnosis with ovarian cancer as being a major contributory factor in his depressive 'breakdown', noting a subsequent sense of 'slippage'. It is important to note however that whilst for some people the causes of depression can have a discernible reason, for others there may be no identifiable factors. This was experienced by Lee Goodgame (Depression Alliance, 2014a) who felt depressed yet bemusedly pointed to the fact that he was happily married, had a nice home and was doing well at work as a self-employed chef.

Natural changes or events can also be attributed to changes in mood. Becoming a parent, especially for the first time is a monumental event in a person's life which has an impact upon all holistic dimensions. There are many new and powerful emotions to cope with as well as major role changes to accommodate. The signs that a person is not coping may not be easily evident because of the expectations that it *will be difficult*. Although this can seem like an empathic attitude to others going through difficult life events, this expectation can actually limit opportunities for support and increase a person's sense of alienation. Cara, a young mother with postnatal depression, felt very isolated and cut off from others and the world around her (Aiken, 2000). She periodically felt hysterical, desperate, exhausted, inadequate, guilty, boring and resentful of others. Such emotions, even though being potentially totally incapacitating, can be regarded dismissively as simply part and parcel of being a new parent with inadequate support subsequently offered:

> Everyone believed that I was coping really well. I had a wonderful way of hiding my true feelings. That made it more difficult because I just wanted to scream and cry in frustration.
>
> Aiken (2000, p. 26)

There is a sense of isolation and disconnectedness from others reflected here echoing Charlotte Perkins Gilman's (1892, p. 16) documentation of her confinement period in *The Yellow Wallpaper*:

> John does not know how much I really suffer … he laughs at me so about this wallpaper.

This semi-autobiographical account continues with describing the narrator's desperation as her mind becomes tormented by the wallpaper's pattern perceiving a woman to be trapped behind it. This clearly symbolises the narrator's stifling, detached and imprisoned experience of confinement.

A particular difficulty concerns the perception that many of the problems experienced by women after childbirth are 'normal'. Certainly some of the diagnostic categories relating to depression are reflected through the disruption to sleep patterns, physical exhaustion and impairment in social, work or other important areas of functioning. Men as well have issues about becoming a parent and taking on the role of fatherhood as illustrated by Rice-Oxley (2012, p. 59) who describes the transition to family life as 'dramatic and a massive change'. This he equates to the profound sense of culture shock experienced on becoming a father and the uncertain expectations upon his parental role.

The sense that 'life is hard' because of changing circumstances or roles can be extended to other experiences such as starting new jobs, changing schools or gaining promotion. It can also relate to external events or distressing news items as reflected by Tim Lott (1996) whose internal fragmentation felt attuned to the simultaneous 'falling apart' of the world around him. The struggle with symptoms, stigma and a reluctance to accept professional help can lead the person experiencing depression to the point of 'breakdown' or crisis. The colloquial term 'nervous breakdown' refers to the point at which life's demands become physically and emotionally overwhelming and individuals are no longer able to cope (Mayo Clinic, 2014). There can be negative connotations as reflected by Solomon (2002) who regarded it as the point where his 'machinery' gave in. This can lead to a viewpoint whereby depressive symptoms are perceived more as a weakness than a justifiable health problem (Yap et al., 2013). Whatever the perspective or feeling, what is important perhaps is the recognition that professional help is required, something which can lead to effective support being engaged.

DIAGNOSIS

> How would you feel if given a diagnosis of depression?

A diagnosis is made by referring symptoms to a set of criteria and gauging their frequency, duration and impact upon a person's functioning (Figure 4.1). The process of diagnosis is complicated and can be subject to a number of errors and problems. As Kokanovic et al. (2013) assert, a better understanding is needed of how people describe, experience, negotiate and participate in the process of diagnosis. It is also crucial to be mindful of what it might be like to be in receipt of a diagnosis of depression. How, for example, are words perceived and understood after being imparted, especially as they can feel terrifying and continue to resonate with people on account of their associations, many of which are perceived negatively. As Rice-Oxley (2012) observed after being presented with a diagnosis of depression, the words used to describe people with mental health problems have a sinister feel about them being commonly associated with lowered expectations, stereotypical presumptions and discriminatory beliefs.

> What are your thoughts about the list of symptoms in Figure 4.1?

A. Five or more of the following symptoms during a 2-week period representing a change from previous functioning:
  - Depressed mood
  - Markedly diminished interest or pleasure in activities
  - Significant weight loss when not dieting or weight gain, or decrease or increase in appetite nearly every day
  - Insomnia or hypersomnia
  - Psychomotor agitation or retardation
  - Fatigue or loss of energy
  - Feelings of worthlessness or excessive or inappropriate guilt
  - Diminished ability to think or concentrate, or indecisiveness
  - Recurrent thoughts of death and suicidal ideation

B. The symptoms cause clinically significant distress or impairment in social, occupational or other important areas of functioning

C. The symptoms are not due to the direct physiological effects of a substance or a general medical condition

Figure 4.1 Criteria for major depressive episode: *DSM-V*. (From American Psychiatric Association, *Diagnostic and Statistical Manual of Mental Disorders*, 5th ed., APA, Washington, DC, 2013.)

TELLING OTHERS

The receipt of a mental health diagnosis can raise concerns around what people feel comfortable about sharing and what the perceived reaction might be. A blogger writing on the Time to Change (2012) website recounts:

> The hardest part of depression is finding a way to tell people ... I tended to inch my way along to a 'full disclosure': How are you? 'I've not been feeling too good', 'Not great', 'I've been better', 'A little down', ... If people still don't get the message then they're a little slow. Then of course there are some who don't want to accept that you are depressed.

This tentative and rather uncertain approach with others is reflected by individuals interviewed about their experience of depression for the Healthtalk online resource. A number of people strove to give the appearance of coping even though struggling with feelings of depression. A common response encountered when initially trying to explain how they felt to friends and family was the suggestion that they were simply stressed or run down:

> On the face of things I was still functioning. I was still coping. I was still able to smile in the right places ... and I didn't then want to appear as if I can't cope, 'Oh my gosh, gosh, no, no, I'm all right, I'm fine really. Yes, you know, I'm fine, yes, yes, yes, yes. Thank God, you know, I'm well'. But inside, it was something completely different.

The need to project an image of 'coping' was seen as being very important to this interviewee because of the feeling of being regarded by others as strong and capable. Depression is commonly perceived to signify vulnerability or failing, something that 'strong' and 'able' people are expected to withstand. The worry about being told to 'pull yourself together' was commonly cited by interviewees as if changing mood states was merely a question of willpower (Healthtalk). These problems can become internalised as part of a person's depressive thoughts with the sense of being weak or pathetic on account of one's inability to cope. The worry about being belittled or dismissed was expressed by Rice-Oxley (2012) who anticipated comments from others that he was merely suffering with a stress-related problem 'like Marcus Trescothick'. This highlights a lack of understanding and sensitivity towards the very real levels of distress and despair being experienced but also fails to acknowledge the fact that Trescothick himself was diagnosed with depression. Rice-Oxley (2012) felt that the only people he felt he could really talk to openly were those in the know, people living with and experiencing depression. This is a commonly expressed feeling and indicates the importance of peer support resources and initiatives such as self-help groups and online discussion forums. The difficulty in talking with others can also be influenced by worries about the impact this might have. As Solomon (2002, p. 69) reflected:

> Depression is hard on friends. You make what by the standards of the world are unreasonable demands on them, and often they don't have the resilience or the flexibility or the knowledge or the inclination to cope.

Such feelings or worries can inhibit or restrict what individuals feel able to share and impact upon one's critical or negative patterns of thinking, as well as keeping people isolated and cut off from others.

> If experiencing depression what do you feel would help through talking with others?

STIGMA

Stigma can be defined as follows:

> A mark of disgrace or infamy; a sign of severe censure or condemnation; a brand.
>
> *Oxford English Dictionary* (2015)

Cooley's *looking glass self* sees one's identity and self-view as being constructed primarily as a result of how others act and respond to us (Cohen, 1982). Stigma is one of the most significant obstacles for those with mental health problems when seeking help from healthcare professionals (Mental Health Foundation, 2015). Clement et al.'s (2015) study, which focused on depression, found that the perceived stigma was a specific factor in creating uncertainty about finding help. This also reflects findings in research by Barney et al. (2006) which found 44% of individuals with depression feeling too ashamed to seek professional help. Sally Brampton (2008), who has personal experience of depression, believes that a physical illness is easier to accept and reflects that we would not say 'pull yourself together' to someone suffering with cancer. The insidious experience of stigma can cause this process to become internalised developing a sense of shame and unacceptance for one's condition (Gilbert, 2004). Marcus Trescothick (2008) felt that suffering from depression was a personal failing, reflecting a sense of inadequacy and was shameful and embarrassing. It created a very real barrier in seeking help and expressing his feelings and thoughts to others. As Chuick et al. (2009) indicate, this negative self-appraisal can be a particular problem for men due to societal expectations around masculinity. This is a major problem, especially given the numbers of men who do not seek help or commit suicide as a response to their inner feelings of despair. It is interesting to note the findings from Horgan and Sweeney's (2010) study which indicates that a large number of young people seek help on the Internet as opposed to face-to-face support because of worries over stigma.

DEPRESSIVE EXPERIENCE

The depressive experience can be related to a number of feelings or manifestations. The elements related in this section are commonly experienced aspects and include polarised experiences such as being unable to feel (numbness) or else being overwhelmed with distressing emotions and feeling suicidal. The depressive experience is also explored in relation to maladaptive attempts by individuals to cope with problems. These include methods to gain relief or distract self from distressing symptoms either through self-medicating with alcohol and drugs or from self-harming behaviours.

REDUCED ACTIVITY AND IMMOBILITY

Problems with inactivity can relate to feelings of apathy, fatigue and motor retardation, all of which will impede individuals in their ability to cope with day-to-day life and attend to self-care needs (Reekum et al., 2005). Motor retardation and apathy are commonly experienced within depression, and the reasons for this can be multifaceted and different for each person. Even activities or tasks which can be perceived as easy may feel overwhelming for those with depression (Williams, 2006). Sylvia Plath's (1963, p. 134) semi-autobiographical narrative *The Bell Jar* details Esther Greenwood's attitude of defeat concerning her self-care:

> The sweaty cotton gave off a sour but friendly smell. I hadn't washed my hair for three weeks ... It seemed so silly to wash one day when I would only have to wash again the next. It made me tired just to think about it. I wanted to do everything once and for all and be through with it.

The constricting sense of inertia can also be related to feelings of uncertainty and fear. Andrew Solomon (2002) describes a feeling of paralysis relating to seemingly simple daily activities such as taking a shower with the mere contemplation filling him with dread. This activity was broken down in his mind into a number of minute details, each with its own set of obstacles and insurmountable challenges. Aoife Inman (Depression Alliance, 2014b) states:

> Depression is far more debilitating than sadness, depression is feeling nothing at all, an inability to construct a future for yourself. It leaves you permanently stationary in time unable to move forwards.

Solomon (2013) accounts for this with the sense of his vitality being swept away, a dynamic regarded by Smith (2013) as being alienated from one's agency, having the knowledge and awareness as to what is required, but being unable to act upon it. The impact can also be noticed in relation to one's communicative ability and level of social interaction. William Styron (1990) found himself struggling to speak with his voice reduced to a faint and wheezy whisper whilst others have described an inability to appropriately animate one's facial expressions (Brosh, 2013).

Elizabeth Wurtzel (1994) describes a particular sense of feeling constantly exhausted, yet being unable to find any relief. She recounted often feeling too tired to think properly or do anything, consequently spending long periods of time in bed unable to get up. This is a common experience with each day's activities feeling totally overwhelming. The state of exhaustion can be physically felt and has been likened by service users as a mental 'stomach bug' (Mulligan, 2014) or flu-like symptoms (Depression Marathon, 2015). The physical manifestation can be such that individuals feel quickly out of breath when engaged in activities or having the sensation of being crushed by a huge weight, all resulting in immobility. This is hard to acknowledge or understand for those who have not experienced depression although the sense of what is experienced can maybe be glimpsed in the following narrative:

> If you're in your bedroom and someone said there's a million dollars on the other side of the room and all you have to do is swing your feet over the edge of the bed, and walk and get the million, you couldn't get the million. I mean you literally couldn't.

Karp (1996, p. 30)

This gets the point across that it is not an issue of willpower or desire but a totally incapacitating and disabling feeling preventing movement or engagement with activities.

DEPRESSION METAPHORS/SIMILES

Personal narratives reveal many different ways in which people seek to represent their depression through figures or concepts. This gives form for what otherwise can feel shapeless or hard to decipher. Perhaps one of the most cited is Churchill's reference to a 'black dog' to represent his dark moods (Breckenridge, 2012). Solomon (2002) illustrated his depression through the example of an oak tree being suffocated by a vine. As previously mentioned, Sylvia Plath's (1963) *The Bell Jar* potently conveys the sense of total alienation and detachment felt. Similarly, Katherine Stone (2007) wrote in her blog about feeling trapped inside a bubble, disconnected from the world around her. The creation of metaphors or similes generally sums up qualities or dynamics from a person's internal experience illustrating what is felt by them. It assists in providing a means for service users and others to comprehend something of what is being experienced. There are a number of different metaphorical concepts reflected with commonly expressed examples relating to loneliness, immobility and alienation (Vatne and Naden, 2012) or staleness, suffocation and sourness (Williams et al., 1990). Another frequently related theme links metaphors with qualities of darkness, for example, 'interminable grey summer' (Brampton, 2008), 'blackness' (Welch, 2010) or an 'all-consuming darkness' (Adams, 2015). The elements of light and dark are reflected by Brampton (2008, p. 291) as representing movement between ill-health and wellness:

> You know the sun is there and you long for it to appear but every morning you wake to a flat, low cloud ... the grey sometimes relieved by a tantalising glimpse of sunlight or a sudden, shockingly blue sky.

Metaphors can also be very evocative of the emotional experience as revealed in Woodgate's (2006) study through examples such as 'vortex of hell' and 'nightmare'. Importantly they can provide a rich and expressive mode for communicating and sharing one's inner experience with others. For a person experiencing depression, the experience of being heard and acknowledged is vital for counteracting pervasive feelings of isolation and loneliness.

> Which of the metaphors expressed here do you feel the most expressive and why?

NUMBNESS/ANHEDONIA

Numbness and anhedonia relate to an inability to *feel* or respond to emotions. The depressive experience can involve a sense of detachment and numbness, in essence an inability to *feel*. The numbing, chilling and detached quality of depression is powerfully symbolised by Plath (1963, p. 250):

> To the person in the bell jar, blank and stopped as a dead baby, the world itself is the bad dream. A bad dream ... maybe forgetfulness, like a kind snow, should numb and cover them.

This sense of numbness is echoed in a number of postings on the Depression Forum with members reflecting their inability to connect emotionally to the world around them. Some individuals even state their longing for feelings such as sadness, with crying providing them with an important release. Similarly, as one Healthtalk (2013) interviewee related:

> I've got no emotions on anything. I don't feel happy I don't feel sad, I've just got the same face on all the time.

Numbed emotions or *not feeling* can be regarded as a self-protective factor, providing a distance from feelings of despair. This brings with it, though, its own problems with individuals longing to regain the capacity to feel. Feeling is an essential human attribute which powerfully defines who we are and connects us to the world in which we live.

A related concept to that of numbness is that of anhedonia which basically refers to a person's inability to feel pleasure and is one of the primary diagnostic criteria for depression (Gorwood, 2008). It can relate to all activities such as social, leisure and sexual and have a significant impact upon a person and their relationships with others. The all-encompassing nature of this experience is reflected by Styron (1990) who recounts the almost total lack of pleasure he felt on receiving a major award (Priz Mondial Cino del Duca) which included a trip to Paris and a £25,000 cheque. Similarly, Elizabeth Wurtzel (1994) writes about her time at college, which should have been the 'time of her life', and being unable to gain any pleasure or excitement from it. Whilst this might be hard to fathom for a number of people it illustrates the potency of depressive symptoms. In these instances individuals note their awareness of the fact that they should be enjoying themselves yet remaining detached from their emotional selves.

HOPELESSNESS AND DESPAIR

A polar opposite to the blankness and numbed emotional response covered in the previous section is the experience of despair, defined by the *Oxford English Dictionary* (2015) as relating to a state of hopelessness. The absence of hope is a devastating and disabling experience leading to inactivity, isolation, pain and thoughts of suicide. Hopelessness can feel like a crushing weight which makes all purposeful movement seem impossible.

Marcus Trescothick (2008) related how completely powerless he felt in tackling his nega-tive thoughts and feelings, being unable to do anything to affect change. These experi-ences, helplessness and disengagement from activities, are defining features of depression (American Psychiatric Association, 2013; Hammen and Watkins, 2008). It will clearly have a further detrimental impact upon one's mood state with a downward spiral hard to avoid. This is reflected by postings across a range of discussion forums which illus-trate the all-pervading nature of hopelessness. There are expressions about being unable to make friends, feel fulfilled or see any hope for change. The inability to socialise or feel connected is even reflected by some when at self-help group meetings with other depressed people. This powerful illustration of hopelessness is matched by postings which apologise in advance to potential readers for wasting their time.

The counter to hopelessness is hope which plays a vital role in helping people recover from depression (Williams, 2012). This vital element can be instilled through engage-ment with healthcare professionals (NICE, 2015), as expressed by Trescothick (2008) who gained the hope and belief that he could be helped. Hope can also be instilled through contact with peers – other people who have experienced depression. This offers a sense of connectedness and understanding as well as vital opportunities for hearing about others' recovery and contemplating possibilities for self. These aspects will be explored further in Section 2: Experiencing support.

FEELING SUICIDAL

The thoughts and feelings present for those contemplating suicide include beliefs about being a burden to others, seeing it as a means of ending one's tormented existence or feel-ing unworthy and not deserving to live (Holmes, 2002). The recorded number of suicides for 2013 in the United Kingdom and ROI was 6708 (Samaritans, 2015). The incidence of suicide is significantly higher for men than women (Department of Health, 2015; ONS, 2015), with prominent issues relating to perceived failings as a provider and protector or a recognition of one's progressive ageing and sense of mortality (Oliffe et al., 2010). Attempting suicide can be a response to feelings that it is the only way to escape from the intensity of intense pain and suffering (Vatne and Naden, 2012). This is reflected by Serani (2011, p. 4) who states:

> At first the mere idea of killing myself brought relief … I didn't bother to con-sider the fallout from what my suicide would do to those who love me either. All I wanted was to be free of the emotional pain.

This highlights how a person's total being can feel permeated with feelings of hopeless-ness, a sense that nothing can be done to elevate one's mood state from the depths of despair. There is also expression here of pain, a devastating and deeply distressing experi-ence which incorporates all holistic dimensions. It is therefore unsurprising to note the increase in suicidal ideation, contemplated as a means of ending and escaping one's tor-mented existence. Thoughts about suicide can be contemplated at length with a meticu-lous degree of planning considered. For Wurtzel (1994), imagining the act of committing suicide even included planning for external details such as the background music she would have playing at the time. The degree of intention to end one's own life will vary significantly for each person. Individuals will also experience their own different range of thoughts and feelings concerning intent. In some cases suicidal thoughts and meticulous plans can provide relief for a person who feels that this is one area of their existence over which they have ultimate control. Alternatively risks of fatality can also arise from ambivalent feelings, self-neglect or the inability to adequately care for self, as recounted by Solomon (2002, p. 69):

> I didn't particularly want to die but I also didn't at all want to live.

A further example is given by Haig (2015) who writes about not wanting to be born as opposed to committing suicide. In many cases these terrifying thoughts occur without anybody else being aware of the internal turmoil a person is experiencing. Tim Lott (1996), for example, contemplated jumping off a high roof, falling under a tube train or asphyxiating himself with car fumes. His thoughts and actions on these occasions had him literally and figuratively teetering on the edge of a precipice with what he regarded as a very serious risk of carrying out these actions. It was pure chance, an abstract thought or a series of random circumstances which prevented him from acting upon his urges. A point worth noting is that the inability of carrying out these actions resulted at the time in a deepening of his internal sense of failure.

Conversely, a factor which can impede suicidal actions is the presence of depression itself. The lack of energy or volition can be a significant factor as reflected by Solomon (2002) who periodically felt too 'dumbly lethargic' to even contemplate suicide. This is subject to changes in mood state and it needs noting that an elevation in emotion can potentially heighten the risk of suicide with individuals having both the energy and volition to act upon their feelings (Gray, 2013). It is a view however which Mittal et al. (2009) challenge stating that it still remains to be substantiated.

An aspect connected with suicidal acts is the perception of it being a 'cry for help' but therefore not a 'real' attempt to kill oneself. This is commonly regarded as an annoying or unwelcome behaviour with those concerned being seen as 'manipulative'. Having thoughts or actions about ending one's life does in itself show a desperate need for help and support. It can at times feel the only way that some people have of reflecting to others how desperate they feel and their urgent need of help (Wurtzel, 1994). It is indeed a terrible tragedy when people actually do end their lives and can leave others bewildered and shocked, sometimes with no real awareness as to the depths of their despair, as for example, with the death of the footballer Gary Speed. This outlines another issue, bereavement through suicide which is a deeply complex and troubling experience leaving others to struggle with their own depressive experience. It also leaves people with a plethora of emotions and unanswered questions, trying to understand what caused someone close to them to take their own life. The sense of bewilderment and seeking for meaning is reflected in a number of narratives or even songs such as Tom Robinson's *Don't Jump Don't Fall* or the Stranglers' *Dagenham Dave*.

It is important to finish this part by illustrating some of the protective agencies involved in suicide prevention or support for those left behind that are highly recommended within personal narratives. These include Survivors of Suicide, CALM, the Samaritans, Papyrus and MayTree. Contact details for these and other agencies are included within Chapter 8.

ISOLATION AND ALIENATION

A major problem encountered by those with depression concerns the feeling that one is alone, and indeed Brampton (2008, p. 1) regards depression as the 'disease of loneliness'. Loneliness and depression coexist, with each element impacting upon the other (Cacioppo et al., 2006). It can affect relationships which in a sense themselves become *depressed* with an increased likelihood of divorce (Harrar and DeMaria, 2006). Narrative accounts show how it becomes harder to form new relationship as well as maintain existing ones with negative and critical self-thinking causing people to isolate themselves away from friends and family (Earl, 2013; Johnstone, 2005). The sense of isolation can also be felt spiritually with the profound experience of being alienated from God, cementing a person's sense of total disconnection (Giesbrecht, 2014). Misinformed attitudes can exacerbate this situation, something experienced by Sally Brampton (2008) who encountered people holding the mistaken belief that she would prefer to be left alone. This probably illustrates difficulties held by others with their uncertainty and discomfort at relating to people with depression. Whilst individuals might periodically choose to be alone it does not mean that this is their constant wish. They can also have very mixed and ambiguous feelings about seeking to be on their own. In any case, isolating oneself can occur because of a number of patterns of thinking such as feeling unworthy, convinced others will be burdened or that one will be rejected. Difficulties with social contact can lead to an active avoidance of other people. This heightens feelings of isolation and disengagement which in turn further reinforce negative patterns of thinking such as feeling unloved (Raymond and DePaulo, 2002). It sets up a negative spiral of thinking resulting in a heightened sense of alienation. Some of these experiences are illustrated in blog postings on the Time to Change website where individuals reflect upon the desperate loneliness in having no-one to confide in and having to cope with problems on their own. A feeling reflected is of being an 'outsider', coupled with the impression that nobody else can understand what a person is experiencing (Emslie et al., 2006). It is also apparent that feelings of separateness and alienation can occur no matter where a person is, in company or on one's own (Erdner et al., 2002). It is a sense portrayed very vividly by Albert Camus (1982) concerning the feeling and state of being an 'outsider'. The sense of losing connection with others and being truly alone is clearly a terrifying experience, reminiscent of our earliest experiences of vulnerability and the fear of abandonment and annihilation (Winnicott, 1962). It is no wonder therefore that feeling attached, heard and engaged with others is cited so highly in connection with interventional approaches such as peer support or psychological therapies. Yalom's (2005) curative factor of *universality*, the sense that 'I am not alone', for example, is regarded as being a vital element within group therapy.

SLEEP DISTURBANCE

> If unable to sleep, how would this affect your thoughts and feelings?

The sense of hopelessness, despair and inability to function experienced with depression are further compounded through the inability to gain temporary relief through sleep.

Sleep can be a longed for and much needed state yet one which remains cruelly out of one's reach. As reflected by Edington (2002, p. 3):

> When you try to unwind at the end of the day you drag yourself to bed. Then what happens? The mind decides to go into overdrive and to have a journey all of its own … It's funny how life always brings the bad and negative thoughts back to you with more detail, and the happy times just come and go in a flash.

Nutt et al. (2008) note the strong association between sleep disturbance and major depression. This includes the difficulty in initiating or maintaining sleep and early morning wakening. There is some debate though concerning cause and effect in relation to how these elements interact with each other (Morawetz, 2003). Sleep disturbances are common in people experiencing depression and heighten physical, psychological and emotional feelings of distress. This can be seen in Rice-Oxley's (2012, p. 174) narrative:

> After two [o'clock], things get wretched. This is when, if you've been doing this night after night you ask those unanswerable questions: why me? What did I do to deserve this?

The early hours can seem an extremely lonely and desperate place to be, left to struggle through one's own ruminations with reduced ability for distraction or in gaining support from others. The preoccupation with the length of time remaining until daylight and the excruciating slow passage of time is powerfully evoked in Plath's (1963, p. 134) *The Bell Jar*:

> I hadn't slept for seven nights. My mother told me I must have slept, it was impossible not to sleep in all that time, but if I slept, it was with my eyes wide open, for I had followed the green, luminous course of the second hand and the minute hand and the hour hand of the bedside clock through their circles and semi-circles, every night for seven nights…

Disturbances of sleep over a prolonged period can be severely distressing and have a huge impact on the quality of life of those who are depressed (Katz and McHomey, 2002). In reviewing people's narratives the term 'sleep disturbance' falls woefully short of encapsulating what is experienced. It needs acknowledging that for some, the depth of despair felt and the inability to find respite can lead them to contemplate suicide or else seek ways of coping through drink or drugs.

COPING WITH DEPRESSIVE FEELINGS: MALADAPTIVE COPING APPROACHES

Although it is important to remember that any kind of coping mechanism is a communication of hope from the person experiencing depression, some coping approaches can become maladaptive. Whilst providing temporary relief these methods are usually not sustainable and ultimately reinforce and heighten difficulties. They are usually self-initiated and contrary to medical advice and include approaches such as self-medicating and self-harming behaviours. Responding to depressive feelings through the use of alcohol or drugs provides a means of gaining respite from emotional, mental and physical pain (Oliffe et al., 2012). This is supported by Brampton (2008) who stated that 'when she drank she didn't *feel*.' Likewise, Welch (2010) relates getting 'legless', not for pleasure but to blot things out. Alcohol initiates chemical changes in the brain which promotes feelings of relaxation, giving a temporary positive impact on mood (Drink Aware, 2015), and therefore, many people who suffer with depression will use alcohol to achieve these feelings. The essence here is about *not feeling* or in achieving relief even if only temporarily from unsettling and distressing emotions. It clearly extends beyond the use of alcohol or drugs to also include smoking, caffeine consumption, sleeping pills, increased activity and exercise. For example, Mendelsohn (2012) found people with a lifetime history of depression being twice as likely to smoke as those not experiencing this condition. Methods and attempts to self-medicate though are common amongst those experiencing depression. Bolton et al. (2009) found up to a quarter of those with mood disorders using alcohol or drugs to relieve symptoms and reduce emotional distress, with men more than twice as likely as women to be affected. Also gaining respite, alcohol or drugs can be regarded as providing individuals with a much desired period of functioning. This is reflected by Gwyneth Lewis (2006) who found that drinking allowed her an escape from her 'normal' life, allowing her to slip into a parallel universe where she could function and move more easily.

There are a number of problems with self-medication including a heightening of depressive symptoms (Gilman and Abraham, 2001) and increased risk of suicide (Sullivan et al., 2005). Despite this, the initial or momentary relief can make this an enticing option which helps to illustrate why relapse rates are so high for those suffering with alcohol problems (Kipping, 2013). Self-medication is about trying to feel better or to suppress one's feelings but it is generally the case that cumulative harm is being caused as a consequence. Other *self-harming* behaviours such as skin cutting can be engaged in to the same end, reducing tension and seeking relief from unwelcome thoughts and feelings (Brain et al., 1998; Briere and Gil, 1998). These particularly occur within states of anxiety and depression with psychological characteristics and stressful life events being contributory factors (Madge et al., 2011). It should be noted though that deliberate self-harm also occurs in non-clinical populations (Klonsky et al., 2003). Skin cutting appears to be the most common method occurring in around 70% of individuals who deliberately self-harm (Langbehn and Pfohl, 1993). The Selfharm UK website includes a large number of postings from young people showing the stress they are under and their self-harming as ways of coping with exam pressures, relationships, depressed feelings and bullying. A common driving factor is the need to distance oneself from problems, thoughts and feelings whereas some postings indicated self-harming being a means of punishing oneself or of pain making a person feel alive. Whatever the self-medicating or self-harming approach used or the effect being sought, such methods do not engage with the underlying cause, the internal feelings of distress. More effective support addressing these internal feelings is needed. This is explored in the following section detailing narrative experiences of receiving help.

If experiencing depression, how hard do you think it might be not self-medicating with any of the approaches noted earlier?

SECTION 2: EXPERIENCING SUPPORT

Interview narratives

I got admitted to hospital and basically they hit me with drugs... They just drugged me out and I was walking about like a zombie.

I did a mindfulness course with a psychologist and it was pretty good at stabilising things ... meditating, ignoring the thoughts.

All they did [in hospital] was sit and observe me and take notes. That really upset me ... I expected a bit more than what they were actually giving me.

I had the full works [ECT], 3 or 4 courses. But it didn't change anything for me.

There [in a secure hospital] they have one on one attention and they work long hours each day. So they build up a rapport and relationship with you.

Talking therapy has got to be the way to go forward ... that would have helped me right from the very start.

My mental health nurse was talking about endorphins and all that and I just didn't want to know about endorphins. So leave the technical stuff out of it, just be there.

Yes I had a couple of friends and a super daughter in law but my husband was absolutely brilliant ... just being there to give me a hug when I needed it.

The best support was from a counsellor.

This section is concerned with the experience of receiving support. It examines the lived and felt experience for those with depression when offered various interventions. The approaches covered in this section include in-patient care, psychological therapies, medication, creative activities and peer support.

TALKING THERAPIES/PSYCHOTHERAPEUTIC INTERVENTIONS

What do you feel people with depression list as the beneficial aspects of psychotherapy?

Psychological or talking therapies have demonstrated equal levels of effectiveness to pharmaceutical interventions in treating mild to moderate depression (Kennedy et al., 2004) or greater effectiveness if offered in combination (Pampallona, 2004). Although only found to be modestly effective with children and adolescents (Weisz et al., 2006), they offer substantial treatment interventions for both younger and older adults (Cuijpers et al., 2009). There are many different types of counselling and psychotherapeutic approaches available. Experiences here can be influenced by many factors such as a therapist's interpersonal skills, number and type of sessions accessed and whether support is offered through individual or group therapy. CBT, for example, is recommended alongside psychodynamic psychotherapy and interpersonal therapy by NICE (2009) and has been found to be effective in improving depressive symptoms and tackling negative behaviours (Kinsella and Garland, 2008). Other approaches such as psychodynamic therapy have been found through research to be beneficial in helping individuals attend to their feelings differently, encouraging resilience and relieving the intensity and duration of depressive episodes (Smith, 2009). A core facilitative element noted was the therapeutic relationship developed with therapists. The importance of this is heightened through the therapist's manner and the sense one gets of feeling secure, acknowledged and supported:

> I don't know exactly what it was, the manner, the tone, the voice, the calm assurance; whatever it was. It was almost like someone putting an arm around you ... I had begun the process of coming back to me.
>
> Trescothick (2008, p. 251)

There are many personal narratives attesting to the transformative and healing power offered through psychotherapy (Fereday, 2014; Klein and Elliott, 2006). The majority of individuals with depression interviewed for the Healthtalk site said that talking therapies had helped them and were regarded as one of the most helpful approaches in treating depression. The psychotherapeutic approaches experienced here included CBT, person-centred counselling, psychosynthesis, systemic consultation, psychodynamic approaches, psychoanalysis, art therapy, group therapy and Gestalt therapy. For many people, what was especially helpful was having the freedom to talk about feelings and thoughts, being able to unburden themselves and gain a greater understanding about their problems. This helped facilitate change, bringing about improvements in their lives. Of particular value was the feeling of being free to talk without the worry of reproachful or critical responses:

> It was a big relief to have someone who I could tell anything I wanted, anything that was bothering me, and not worry about what they might think about it or how it might affect our relationship.

This is vitally important, having a place of expression for one's thoughts and feelings as well as being heard and acknowledged. This was related by a blogger concerning the sense of feeling validated by her therapist, thereby empowered to get on with her life (Time to Change, 2014a). Another blogger documented the sense of hope her therapist instilled in her, a vital element which helped foster a sense of self-sufficiency and resilience blogger (Time to Change, 2014b). These narratives highlight some crucial elements relating to the psychotherapeutic process concerning opportunities to express oneself and feel heard, making sense of one's thoughts and feelings, as well as the absolutely essential element, the instillation of hope. What is concerning is the number of people unable to access psychotherapeutic approaches despite a wish for this type of intervention. Indeed, amongst the treatments most often cited as missed out on are counselling and psychotherapy

(Mind, 2003). This indicates a very important need with a number of individuals feeling insufficiently supported despite the Improving Access to Psychological Therapies (IAPT) initiative (DoH, 2012) and the 4-year plan of action (DoH, 2011).

A further element to consider with regard to psychological therapies involves self-help guides. Two notable examples developed for use with depression relate to *Overcoming Depression* (Gilbert, 2009) which uses CBT techniques and *The Mindful Way through Depression* (Williams et al., 2007), which utilises the mindfulness approach. Both of these titles receive favourable reviews from people with depression on Amazon. There is a size-able market for self-help guides although the available titles are clearly of very variable quality.

MEDICATION

NICE (2009) advise against using antidepressants as a routine approach to treat mild depression because of the poor risk–benefit ratio. However, with moderate to severe depression they propose medication as a potential intervention to offer alongside psychological therapies. Selective serotonin reuptake inhibitors (SSRIs) appear to be their preferred choice of medication, regarded as having equal effectiveness to other antidepressants but with a more favourable risk–benefit ratio. Other groups of anti-depressant include serotonin–noradrenaline reuptake inhibitors (SNRIs) and the less used tricyclic antidepressants (TCAs) and monoamine oxidase inhibitors (MAOIs). A particular issue encountered by those required to take medication concerns having to reorientate one's identity (Garfield et al., 2003), which can include an affirmation of being a person who has a stigmatised disorder (Karp, 1996). As Solomon (2002) experienced, this feeling was increased by the 'expressions of horror' he received from others after revealing that he would have to continue taking medication indefinitely. Research findings generally show adherence with antidepressant medication to be poor (Bosworth et al., 2008; Navarro, 2010) with one of the main factors relating to troubling side effects (Mark et al., 2009). Participants in Kikuchi et al.'s (2012) study listed side effects as sexual dysfunction, fatigue, dry mouth, weight gain, sweating, tremor and drowsiness. In a study examining the impact from SSRI medication, par-ticipants reported a reduction in positive emotions, being emotionally detached or disconnected, and feeling like a 'zombie' or 'robot' (Price et al., 2009). An important aspect here concerns the findings that adverse side effects can contribute to an abrupt discontinuation and non-compliance with antidepressant medication (Ashton et al., 2005). Although side effects raise particular concerns, Bull et al.'s (2002) study indi-cated that continuation with medication is increased through discussing potential side effects when prescribing. This is important as increased compliance with medica-tion can reduce the risk of relapse (Katon et al., 2001). The impact from side effects can be profoundly unsettling causing acute distress and significantly impacting upon a person's life. Studies demonstrate that antidepressants are associated with sexual dysfunction in a substantial proportion of people (Baldwin, 2013). Clearly, this will impact upon self-esteem as well as a person's relationships with others. Whilst sexual difficulties during antidepressant treatment often resolve as depressive symptoms lift, they can endure over long periods and for some individuals persist indefinitely

(Bahrick and Harris, 2009). A key issue to consider concerns the balance between positive results and troubling side effects. An interviewee in Karp's (1996, p. 96) work stated:

> It made my mood brighter but I hated the side effects.

This raises the issue of 'pay off', weighing up the inconvenience or distress caused against the benefits which can be profoundly felt. The experience of taking medication can feel consoling through the framing of one's problems as a treatable chemical disorder. It can also provide hope and bring relief for torturous feelings and thoughts (Karp, 1996). This desire for relief can be a strong motivator to commence medication as expressed in the 'Depression Alliance' (2014c) blog which illustrates an individual's desperate need to feel better, initially unconcerned about potential side-effects. It illustrates the sense of longing for some respite from troubling symptoms. Discussion threads on the Patient forum illustrate a number of shared experiences with posts comparing side effects and experiences of changing medication or reducing dosages. There was also a significant issue of waiting for beneficial effects to be felt. A blogger describes her frustration about the lack of immediate relief felt from her medication despite doctors increasing the dose (Piggot, 2011). This is a feeling expressed through numerous personal narratives such as Styron's (1990) unbearable and torturous wait for his new medication to become effective. When it does work though the experience can feel transformative as expressed by Wurtzel (1994) regarding the wonderful moment when her medication finally 'kicked in' and she was able to get out of bed. Improvements can be gradually felt over time or in some cases suddenly, with brighter feelings experienced as a revelation:

> There is a pigeon cooing on the balcony outside my bedroom. It is pleasant and soothing. I haven't noticed birdsong for a long time ... I feel strange in that I feel normal ... I know quite clearly and calmly now, like a camera suddenly finding focus, that I really have been ill, and equally that I have begun to recover.
>
> Lott (1996, p. 245)

When medication does not alleviate symptoms though, even after waiting for weeks it can feel unbearable, something Sally Brampton (2008, p. 20) described as

> almost more catastrophic ... than the illness itself.

The worry here was that if modern medicine could not cure her, then what could, showing how easily hope can be lost. The findings that antidepressant use significantly improves depressive symptoms after 3 months of treatment for between 50% and 65% of people (Royal College of Psychiatrists, 2015b) will be hard for those not helped.

Evidently, individual experiences with antidepressant medication are very different and unique to each person. The concerns of a number of people posting on the Depression Forum were that they would struggle to function without medication. It is apparent that the experiences of taking medication differ vastly and that each individual has their own individual story to relate.

IN-PATIENT CARE

There are times for some people when the support and help needed can only effectively be provided during a period of hospitalisation. This can occur on a voluntary or involuntary basis and for varying time spans. The experience of receiving in-patient care will evoke very mixed feelings amongst those concerned. First, even though care facilities have changed considerably from the institutional environment of bygone years, notions of an earlier culture can still prevail within societal imaginings:

> The acute mental health unit. How these words shame me, for I am now a designated other, a crazy person. Even as I trudge towards the hospital, I feel disgusted by the idea that I am entering the cuckoo's nest.
>
> Lott (1996, p. 242)

This is not an isolated feeling with a number of other narratives picking up on the associated stigma and disquiet associated with mental healthcare facilities. The 'Cuckoo's Nest' mentioned here relates to a very powerful and iconic representation which still resonates powerfully decades after Kesey's (1962) book and Douglas and Forman's (1975) film entered into the public arena. Admission to a mental health facility does therefore cause difficulties for people if feeling too ashamed to tell others (Brampton, 2008). The nature of one's admission to hospital can also be a significant factor with involuntary admission (sectioning) having strong stereotypical and stigmatising associations. As illustrated by postings on The Sites discussion forum, fears and uncertainties can be experienced by those being admitted concerning their fantasies and expectations about the risk posed by their fellow 'patients'. Whilst these fears were generally unrealised, experiences in hospital were very varied with some receiving good support from staff and others feeling unsupported and inadequately supervised. There was a strong sense communicated about the prevailing sense of boredom and apathy with a lot of time spent smoking. This differing experience of involuntary hospital care is reflected amongst participants in Hughes et al.'s (2009) qualitative study. Some respondents cited generally positive experiences with effective support received from mental health staff and fellow patients. Others however expressed negative aspects in relation to their experience with medication and their relationships with healthcare professionals.

The importance of timely hospital admission is reflected by Samantha (DBSA, 2015) who requested help after her depressive symptoms worsened and she felt suicidal:

> Being hospitalized was one of the scariest things I ever did, but looking back on it now, I believe it was really what I needed. I not only needed medication and a safe place, but I needed some intensive therapy, some ideas of ways to release some feelings.

The narrative here clearly acknowledges the concept of *asylum*, a refuge or place of safety where one can feel secure and receive much needed support. This is reflected by a number of interviewees in Karp's (1996) study who described hospital as a true asylum providing them relief and allowing them to 'crash'. It can also provide momentarily relief from having to maintain the pretence to others that everything is 'normal' and offers dramatic evidence that support is needed (Wurtzel, 1994). A further aspect raised by Samantha (DBSA, 2015) was the fact that she had to fight to get admitted, an aspect which is worryingly echoed by a number of contributors for the Healthtalk online resource. Narratives here acknowledged having to 'act up' to secure admission despite experiencing very acute feelings of depression. Shortages within the available bed provision can mean that some people have to wait longer to receive this type of help and are liable to being more acutely unwell. This can be significant as the 'climate' one enters can have a strong impact, something related through a number of personal accounts as being a devastating and terrifying experience leaving individuals feeling like damaged goods. Clearly, being around other acutely unwell people can be scary but will also impact upon how individuals subsequently view and define themselves as a consequence. This illustrates the need to acknowledge some of the difficulties and issues people may have with this experience, provide sensitive and effective support and make appropriate environmental changes.

ECT

What are your thoughts about ECT as a treatment intervention for depression?

ECT is a strongly debated treatment intervention and one which generates a significant degree of unrest. This in part is caused by memorable scenes in the film *One Flew Over the Cuckoo's Nest* (Douglas and Forman, 1975) where this intervention is shown being used for social control and punishment as opposed to therapeutic purposes. The treatment itself involves passing an electrical current through the brain to produce an epileptic fit and is used if a person

- Has severe, life-threatening depression
- Has not responded to medication or talking treatments
- Has found it helpful in the past
- Is experiencing a manic episode which is severe or is lasting a long time
- Is catatonic
- Has severe postnatal depression (Royal College of Psychiatrists, 2015c)

It is generally seen as an effective treatment modality for severe depression as evidenced by the ECT Accreditation Service who conducted a survey between September 2004 and February 2006. They found the following:

- 72% of service users said that ECT had been helpful.
- 20% said that it had had no effect.
- 5% said they would not want it again.
- 14% believed that it had changed or saved their lives (Mind, 2013a).

Narrative accounts around the effectiveness of ECT vary as observed in discussion threads on the Depression Forum. These illustrate a number of fears held by individuals with frequent mention of the 'Cuckoo's Nest' and memory loss. This can be countered by a number of personal accounts such as Juliet's (Beyond Blue, 2014) which praises ECT as a beneficial treatment method. Similarly, blogger Vicarious Therapy (2010) recounted how miraculous ECT seemed after receiving a 13th ECT treatment, having initially been feeling close to suicide but subsequently excited and pleased to be alive.

These narratives are certainly encouraging although need to be viewed in relation to accounts where it has not been effective or has produced troubling or distressing effects. The painter Lawrence Lee (2007), who spent almost $10,000 for his ECT treatments, recounted:

> For some five months following the ECT treatments I felt better, but I had lost something in the process. I had somehow detached from the wellspring of ideas that had been my creative salvation for decades.
>
> Lee (2007, p. 181)

Other detrimental effects are related by interviewees on the Healthtalk website who expressed feeling 'woozy' and completely disoriented and losing memories. Memory loss in particular can be particularly distressing with one interviewee recounting losing up to 7 years of her memory including the birth of her son. Tracy, another interviewee felt that ECT did nothing for her except remove her memory, an intervention she regarded as barbaric. Another powerful narrative expressing the problems caused through loss of memory is shown in Box 4.1.

The various narrative accounts available illustrate some fairly polarised opinions ranging from 'life-saving' to 'traumatic' and 'abusive'. It does not work for everyone and can produce some troubling and distressing side effects, particularly memory

---

Box 4.1 ECT and memory loss

At work was I then a disgrace?

From this hole in my mind – is this great space?

For I found, to my shame,

This face – what's his name?

Or this name – who's got the right face?

Who began this outrageous farce?

Who decides to switch on and pass?

A current designed

To 'repair' this bent mind?

Do they really know elbow from arse?

Source: Extract from Vincent, R., Early closing Thursday, in: Carver, N. et al., eds., *Greater Goings On … (Than You Would Ever Guess …)*, Asylum Publishing, Sheffield, England, 2007, p. 43.

loss. For those it does work for though the effects can facilitate a return to coping and functioning day to day.

CREATIVE OUTLETS

What benefits do you feel can be gained by people experiencing depression through creative outlets?

A valuable mode of coping with depressive symptoms includes having an outlet for self-expression as provided by various creative or artistic modes. Rachel Kelly (2014) writes about the healing power of poetry which helped her to cope and recover from severe depression. It is a very expressive medium which can symbolise thoughts and feelings in a very powerful way and provides an important outlet for emotions. Another creative medium offering a rich and valuable means of externalising emotions is art. An example of its positive qualities is illustrated by Sandum (Depression Alliance, 2014d) who writes about how it provided him with a lifeline and a means of coping with unbearable pain:

> When I feel overwhelmed with misery and go to my studio, I can regain some form of control by painting. This is how I've been able to survive...Depression screams that you're alone and nobody understands. But when I look at any painting by Van Gogh, all of that doubt disappears. Vincent feels my pain. It is in every brushstroke.

This narrative expresses the sense of connection and acknowledgement realised through observing others' work. This can no doubt feel very heartening with the sense that one's inner feelings and torment are shared and connected with. This reflects what many people feel in relation to, for example, a musician's song lyrics, a writer's characterisation or a poet's lyrical prose. Creative modes such as art can provide an important function of enabling communication for times when speaking is too difficult, which as shown within a personal narrative enables one to be heard (Mind, 2013b). The narratives detailed earlier highlight how vital engaging in artistic endeavours such as poetry and art can be for one's own sense of coping. This sees artistic modes as providing conduits through which distressing emotions can be channelled. It reflects a process regarded by the famous German writer and playwright Goethe (Boerner, 2015) as essential, enabling him to come to terms with whatever was troubling him through drawing or writing and helping to create a sense of inner peace.

In Van Lith et al.'s (2011) study service users described art making as a transformative activity enabling them to take greater control of their lives, resulting in feeling stronger, more confident and more capable of driving their journey of recovery. It is evident that these benefits can be achieved through a very diverse range of creative activities with each person finding their own outlet. A Depression Alliance (2014e) blogger for example described how knitting brought her relief from negative patterns of thinking through the creation of something beautiful.

> The reason knitting is such a therapeutic activity for me is that it allows me to create something. No matter how I am feeling at the time I start knitting, I am reminded that I am releasing content into the world and that the content I am releasing is beautiful.

Another creative mode of coping is illustrated in Erin's (2015) blog 'Daises and Bruises' about her experience with depression. It includes a fascinating feature about her *good things jar*, a painted jar within which she stores bits of paper with all the good things that happen to her in the course of a year written down. She reflected that whenever she had done this it helped her to feel better about her day however bad it might have been. It did not stop her having negative experiences although helped by changing how she thought about and processed them. Similarly, Clare Law (Depression Alliance, 2014f) records the best features of each day in her blog 'Three Beautiful Things'. She reflected that some tiny joys can seem so insignificant such as pansies growing between a wall and the pavement that they would be forgotten if not deliberately contemplated. The collective items documented had a cumulative effect and helped to maintain her mood. The Dealing with Depression Forum includes a section called the Home Straight which features stories about beating depression. The postings showcase a multitude of experiences and approaches which have elevated mood and helped individuals to cope. The feel of the site is very supportive and safe with those posting information mindful of potential triggers for others and writing messages of support and pleasure at others' recovery. The value of resources such as these concerns the sense of engagement felt as well as the gaining of hope and ideas from what is being shared. Clearly the range of creative activities will be wide including examples as diversely different as sport, cooking, playing music or embroidery.

PEER SUPPORT

This section examines the very significant benefits and support received from peers, others who have personal experience of depression. This includes online and face-to-face self-help groups and family and friends. The key element here relates to feelings of connectedness, acceptance and understanding which are fostered. Mike Bush has family experience with suicide and has campaigned for more effective peer support to be provided to loss survivors (Kembe, 2013). His work has been instrumental in the development of professional guidelines and the creation of a range of crisis services and peer-led resources and initiatives. This acknowledges the value that that renewed engagement with others has in tackling feelings of disconnectedness, isolation and hopelessness, all common experiences with depression. Haig (2015) expresses the feeling that *nobody understands* being countered by the realisation that in fact many people have experienced and are experiencing related difficulties. This acknowledgement can be enormously consoling in that

> Understanding that we are not alone and hearing other people express similar thoughts and feelings is quite possibly the best pain relief there is.
>
> Brampton (2008, p. 259)

This stresses the essential need for peer engagement, which can be attained through a variety of means including self-help groups or online blogs and discussion forums. Self-help groups in particular offer a number of beneficial aspects to those with depression:

> I felt really great to be surrounded by people who spoke my language. Because when I'm talking to the therapist, it's him there and me here the patient. But in this group I felt that we were more equal, you know because we all had gone through the same thing.

> Healthtalk (2015)

The *language* indicated here can perhaps be regarded as the *language of depression*, expressive communication of inner feelings which are connected with by others who have shared experience. A particular quality of online discussion forums is the provision of a safe and anonymous resource within which to share thoughts and feelings (Parikh and Huniewicz, 2015). They aid recovery through offering hope (Lakeman and Fitzgerald, 2008) and fostering a sense of connection with others (Widemalm and Hjarthag, 2015), which challenge the isolatory sense of having to face this experience alone. Relaying stories about coping and survival have been crucially helpful in counteracting suicidal ideation (Mehlum, 2000). The value of this type of peer support resource is highlighted by a posting on the Dealing with Depression website:

> I stumbled across [this] website. It was a lifeline. I could finally talk to people about how exactly I felt without fear, explain not worry about how they would react to how I was feeling, what I wanted to do.

The comment here illustrates that this is a resource where individuals can express even their most distressing thoughts and receive support and understanding, not rejection or stigma. A notable feature of discussion forums concerns the reciprocal position which individuals engage, both requesting support as well as offering it to others. This recognises the 'experts by experience' descriptor afforded people by nature of their contextual understanding. Helping others can provide individuals with a sense of purpose, value and appreciation. A Time to Change (2014c) blogger relates the benefits she has received through acting as a Time to Change champion, helping to transform her own and others' lives as well as helping to challenge attitudes and promote understanding.

The focus within this section can also be widened to encompass family and friends. The Healthtalk resource shows that despite many initial fears about sharing one's experience of depression with others, many narratives illustrate how family members, friends, neighbours and colleagues were able to understand and be supportive. There was also surprise (and comfort) from learning about the experience of depression from people known to them. These narratives reflected various ways in which support was received in some cases with others simply being available and not necessarily having to say anything. There were also preferences detailed about what is felt as supportive such as being encouraging as opposed to persuading, listening without trying to provide solutions as well as periodically offering a means of distraction.

SECTION 3: LIVING WELL

> ### Interview narratives
>
> *I feel I'm making a bit of a contribution to the students' learning because I can use my experience and they can get a bit of knowledge about it.*
>
> *I set up a work scheme in the area I lived to offer activities and support for older people and joined the Time to Change campaign.*
>
> *I think it [my experience] gave me a better understanding of mental health.*
>
> *I want to give something back … I want to work in mental health and try and help people through support working or counselling.*
>
> *I'm much more aware that people sometimes need somebody to talk to.*
>
> *It's not a weakness to admit that you can't cope with mental health problems. Not being able to cope is not a weakness.*
>
> *I still go a wee bit into that world. I can feel it there as if it's beside me trying to drag me back in. I'm not going and that's it.*

To what degree do you feel it is possible to live well with depression?

As outlined throughout this chapter, the meaning for each person concerning the experience of living with depression will be completely unique with differing views related by each person consulted. There will also be a changing experience concerning the point at which narratives are collected within a person's journey with depression. Asking someone to describe meaning when in the depth of suicidal distress will be very different to asking the same question when they are in recovery, a point at which greater resilience and hope are fostered. It is also a place where individuals report having greater clarity of thought and the ability to accept and accommodate their depressive experience. Here, depression can be regarded as part of one's identity or makeup. As related by Trisha Goddard (NHS Choices, 2014):

> My depression hasn't gone away, but I've learned to live with it … I'm no longer a victim of the illness. Instead, I'm a survivor.

The concept of survivor illustrates a redefining of self, recognising the possession of enhanced resilience and feeling able to live well, even in the presence of depression. Andrew Solomon (2002) welcomes the person he has become as a consequence of his experience with depression. It is a sentiment which is shared by a number of narratives whereby individuals celebrate their personal growth and heightened awareness. The changes noted can also be linked to new learning and personal development:

> I believe that depression is actually a gift. That if we can befriend it, if we can travel with it, that it is showing us things.

Karp (1996, p. 104)

The 'things' that depression can show one can relate to both internal and external dynamics. This involves developing a greater understanding of self and a developed appreciation of relationships, experiences and the world around one. As Gardiner (2002, p. 8) reflects:

> There is nothing like a serious bout of depression to make you take stock. I've had to re-evaluate, re-think and re-design my life right down to the basics.

The experience of depression here can be seen as the catalyst for change although is obviously dependent upon personal circumstances and available support.

For some people an elevation in feelings can be perceived as a sense of 'awakening' with one's perceptual awareness being heightened. An example of this can be seen in interviewees' narratives on the Healthtalk online site which includes the reflection:

> The sun seems to shine better, the colours of nature are much sharper.

This shows not only an appreciation of one's external world but also a sense of fulfilment and enjoyment.

The various factors cited by service users as being important in their recovery process include hope, self-identity, meaning in life and personal responsibility (Mood Café, 2015). These elements highlight some vital factors in helping to promote change and maintain well-being. The sense of transformation is reflected through many individuals' narratives. Sophie Hunt (2015) reflects upon her battle with depression and feels that she triumphed and developed into a more empathic and understanding person. This highlights developing characteristics for coping and a more optimistic view of the future. A blogger writes:

> There is a long road in front of me but, with support from family and friends, I am almost certain I can recover and live a long and healthy life.
>
> Time to Change (2015)

This underlines an element which is crucial and vitally needed by people with depression – *hope* (see Box 4.2). Hope can be kindled even within a backdrop of extreme despair and suicidal ideation as reflected by Julie Hersh (2011). Her narrative details an arduous journey through excruciating feelings of depression to a point of self-resilience and coping. It illustrates that depression can be devastating, totally alienating and draining but can also be enriching, educational and a catalyst for change. Such examples are crucial for those with depression to relate to and to encourage a climate of greater openness and sharing around mental health experience. Kevan Jones, a labour MP, emulated the Norwegian Prime Minister Kjell Magne Bondevik in publicly speaking about his depression in Parliament to which he received an overwhelmingly positive response (Gekoski and Broome, 2014). This prompted sharing from other people about their own related experiences, many of whom he felt were the last people he might have imagined would suffer with depression. It is evident that engaging with others and sharing experiences of depression allows individuals to feel acknowledged and connected. This fits in with peer support opportunities or health promotional initiatives such as the campaigning work of Time to Change and other mental health advocacy groups. It provides opportunities for expressing personal narratives around recovery from depression as well as connecting with others who are sharing their stories.

Box 4.2 Recovery

I feel myself growing stronger.

The scars have begun to heal.

I know that one day with hope and love

The past is not all I will feel.

I'm not going to let you win, rule my life no more.

I will be a stronger person and leave the past behind.

I will start a new chapter,

Despite what's happened to me,

I will fulfil my dreams and hopes, because you can't take them away from me.

Source: Sewell, A., Mine to keep, in: Carver, N. et al., eds., *Greater Goings On ...* (*Than You Would Ever Guess ...*), Asylum Publishing, Sheffield, UK, 2007, p. 26.

The aspects covered in this section show that with timely and effective support tailored appropriately for each person, opportunities to take control of one's own life and develop adaptive coping skills are enabled. With hope kindled and positive coping skills maintained, ways can be found to overcome or coexist with depression.

REFERENCES

Adams, J. (2015). Depression: An all-consuming darkness. https://tuxedage.wordpress.com.

Aiken, C. (2000). *Surviving Post Natal Depression.* Jessica Kingsley Publishers: London, UK.

Amazon. (2015). Customer reviews. www.Amazon.co.uk, accessed 16 April, 2015.

American Psychiatric Association (2013). *Diagnostic and Statistical Manual of Mental Disorders* (5th ed.). APA: Washington, DC.

Ashton, A., Jamerson, B.D., Weinstein, W.L. and Wagoner, C. (2005). Antidepressant-related adverse effects impacting treatment compliance: Results of a patient survey. *Current Therapeutic Research.* 66(2), 96–106.

Bahrick, A.S. and Harris, M.M. (2009). Sexual side effects of antidepressant medications: An informed consent accountability gap. *Journal of Contemporary Psychotherapy.* 39(2), 135–143.

Baldwin, D. (May 2013). Sexual side effects of antidepressant drugs. Paper presented at the *Meeting of Scandinavian College of Neuropsychopharmacology,* Copenhagen, Denmark.

Barney, L.J., Griffiths, K.M., Jorm, A.F. and Christensen, H. (2006). Stigma about depression and its impact on help-seeking intentions. *Australian and New Zealand Journal of Psychiatry.* 40(1), 51–54.

Beyond Blue (2014). Online Forums. https://www.beyondblue.org.au, accessed 17 May, 2015.

Beyond Blue (2015). Depression: Signs and symptoms. http://www.beyondblue.org.au, accessed 3 May, 2015.

Boerner, P. (2015). *Goethe (Life and Times)*. Haus Publishing: London, UK.

Bolton, J.M., Robinson, J. and Sareen, J. (2009). Self-medication of mood disorders with alcohol and drugs in the national epidemiologic survey on alcohol and related conditions. *Journal of Affective Disorders*. 115(3), 367–375.

Bosworth, H.B., Voils, C.I., Potter, G. and Steffens, D.C. (2008). The effects of antidepressant medication adherence as well as psychosocial and clinical factors on depression outcome among older adults. *International Journal of Geriatric Psychiatry*. 23(2), 129–134.

Brain, K.L., Haines, J. and Williams, C.L. (1998). The psychophysiology of self-mutilation: Evidence of tension reduction. *Archives of Suicide Research*. 4, 227–242.

Brampton, S. (2008). *Shoot the Damn Dog*. Bloomsbury Publishing PLC: London, UK.

Breckenridge, C. (2012). Finest Hour. http://www.winstonchurchill.org.

Briere, J. and Gil, E. (1998). Self-mutilation in clinical and general population samples: Prevalence, correlates, and functions. *American Journal of Orthopsychiatry*. 68, 609–620.

Brosh, A. (2013). Depression. http://hyperboleandahalf.blogspot.co.uk.

Brown, C., Connere, K.O., Copeland, V.C., Grote, N., Beach, S., Battista, D. and Reynolds, C.F. (2010). Depression, stigma, race and treatment seeking behaviour and attitudes. *Journal of Community Psychology*. 38(3), 350–368.

Bull, S.A., Hu, H., Hunkeler, E.M., Lee, J.Y., Ming, E.E., Markson, L.E. and Fireman, B. (2002). Discontinuation of use and switching of antidepressants: Influence of patient-physician communication. *The Journal of the American Medical Association*. 288(1), 1403–1409.

Cacioppo, J., Hughes, M., Waite, L., Hawkley, L. and Thisted, R. (2006). Loneliness as a specific risk factor for depressive symptoms: Cross-sectional and longitudinal analysis. *Psychology and Aging*. 21(1), 140–151.

Camus, A. (1982). *The Outsider*. Penguin: London, UK.

Chuick, C.D., Greenfeld, J.M., Greenberg, S.T., Shepard, S.J., Cochran, S.V. and Haley, J.T. (2009). A qualitative investigation of depression in men. *Psychology of Men & Masculinity*. 10(4), 302–313.

Clement, S., Schauman, O., Graham, T., Maggioni, F., Evans-Lacko, S., Bezborodovs, N. et al. (2015). What is the impact of mental-health related stigma on help seeking? A systematic review of quantitative and qualitative studies. *Psychological Medicine*. 45(1), 11–27.

Cohen, M. (1982). *Charles Horton Cooley and the Social Self in American Thought*. Garland: New York.

Cuijpers, P., Van Straten, A., Smit, F. and Andersson, G. (2009). Is psychotherapy for depression equally effective in younger and older adults? A meta-regression analysis. *International Psychogeriatrics*. 21(1), 16–24.

DBSA (2015). Personal narrative. www.dbsalliance.org, accessed 28 October, 2015.

Dealing with Depression Forum. (2015). Forum. http://www.dealingwithdepression.co.uk, accessed 8 July, 2015.

Department of Health (2011). Talking therapies: A four-year plan of action. HMSO: London, UK.

Department of Health (2012). IAPT three-year report. The first million patients. HMSO: London, UK.

Department of Health [DoH] (2015). Suicide prevention: Second annual report. DoH: London, UK.

Depression Alliance (2014a). There must be something wrong with me. http://www.depressionalliance.org, accessed 16 April, 2015.

Depression Alliance (2014b). Does everyone else have their life mapped out? http://www.depressionalliance.org, accessed 1 August, 2015.

Depression Alliance (2014c). Five things I didn't expect from anti-depressants. http://www.depressionalliance.org, accessed 17 May, 2015.

Depression Alliance (2014d). Why art is my lifeline. http://www.depressionalliance.org/, accessed 28 October, 2015.

Depression Alliance (2014e). Why knitting is my therapy. http://www.depressionalliance.org/, accessed 26 October, 2015.

Depression Alliance (2014f). Three beautiful things. http://www.depressionalliance.org, accessed 4 February, 2015.

Depression Forum. (2015). http://www.depressionforums.org, accessed 16 April, 2015.

Depression Marathon (2015). Depression marathon blog. http://depressionmarathon.blogspot.co.uk, accessed 17 May, 2015.

Douglas, M. and Forman, M. (1975). *One Flew Over the Cuckoo's Nest*. United Artists: United States.

Drink Aware (2015). Alcohol and mental health. https://www.drinkaware.co.uk.

Earl, R. (2013). *My Mad Fat Diary*. Hodder & Stoughton: London, UK.

Edington, C. (2002). A day with severe depression. In R. Ramsay, A. Page, T. Goodman and D. Hart (Eds.), *Changing Minds* (pp. 3–6). Gaskell: London, UK.

Emslie, C., Ridge, D., Ziebland, S. and Hunt, K. (2006). Men's account of depression: Reconstructing or resisting hegemonic masculinity? *Social Science & Medicine*. 62(9), 2246–2257.

Erdner, A., Nyström, M., Severinsson, E. and Lützén, K. (2002). Psychosocial disadvantages in the lives of persons with long term mental illness living in a Swedish community. *Journal of Psychiatric and Mental Health Nursing*. 9, 457–463.

Erin (2015). Good Things Jar. http://daisiesandbruises.com, accessed 18 October, 2015.

Fereday, S. (2014). *A Personal Journey through Psychotherapy: A Case Study Revisited*. Karnac Books: London, UK.

Ferrari, A., Charlson, F., Norman, R., Patten, S., Freedman, G., Murray, C. et al. (2013). Burden of depressive disorders by country, sex, age, and year: Findings from the global burden of disease study 2010. *PLOS Medicine*. 10, e1001547.

Gardiner, L. (2002). Resistance is useless. In R. Ramsay, A. Page, T. Goodman and D. Hart (Eds.), *Changing Minds* (pp. 7–8). Gaskell: London, UK.

Garfield, S.F., Smith, F. and Francis, S. (2003). The paradoxical role of antidepressant medication-returning to normal functioning while losing the sense of being normal. *Journal of Mental Health* 12(5), 521–553.

Gekoski, A. and Broome, S. (2014). *What's Normal Anyway? Celebrities Own Stories of Mental Illness*. Constable: London, UK.

Giesbrecht, M. (2014). Depression story. http://www.thoughts-about-god.com/.

Gilbert, P. (2004). Shame, stigma and the family: Skeletons in the cupboard' and the role of shame. In A. Crisp (Ed.), *Every Family in the Land: Understanding Prejudice and Discrimination against People with Mental Illness* (pp. 123–128). Royal Society of Medicine Press Ltd.: London, UK.

Gilbert, P. (2009). *Overcoming Depression: A Self-Help Guide Using Cognitive Behavioural Techniques.* Robinson: London, UK.

Gilman, C.P. (1892). *The Yellow Wallpaper.* Dover Publications: New York.

Gilman, S. and Abraham, H. (2001). A longitudinal study of the order of onset of alcohol dependence and major depression. *Drug and Alcohol Dependence.* 63(3), 277–286.

Gorwood, P. (2008). Neurobiological mechanisms of anhedonia. *Dialogues in Clinical Neuroscience.* 10(3), 291–299.

Gray, C. (2013). Assessment of the suicidal patient in the emergency department. In L.S. Zun (Ed.), *Behavioural Emergencies for the Emergency Physician* (pp. 60–68). Cambridge University Press: Cambridge, UK.

Haig, M. (2015). *Reasons to Stay Alive.* Canongate Books: London, UK.

Hammen, C. and Watkins, E. (2008). *Depression* (2nd ed.), Psychology Press: Hove, East Sussex, England.

Harrar, S. and DeMaria, R. (2006). *Seven Stages of Marriage: Laughter, Intimacy, and Passion Today, Tomorrow and Forever.* Reed Elsevier Inc.: London, UK.

Healthtalk. (2015). http://www.healthtalk.org, accessed 16 April, 2015.

Healthtalk (2013). Depression and low mood. http://www.healthtalk.org, accessed 6 March, 2015.

Hersh, J. (2011). *Struck by Living: From Depression to Hope.* Brown Books Publishing Group: Dallas, TX.

Holmes, J. (2002). *Ideas in Psychoanalysis: Depression.* Icon Books: Cambridge, UK.

Horgan, Á. and Sweeney, J. (2010). Young students' use of the Internet for mental health information and support. *Journal of Psychiatric and Mental Health Nursing.* 17(2), 117–123.

Hughes, R., Hayward, M. and Finlay, W.M.L. (2009). Patients' perceptions of the impact of involuntary inpatient care on self, relationships and recovery. *Journal of Mental Health.* 18(2), 152–160.

Hunt, S. (2015). Why depression can be a gift. http://www.depressionalliance.org/.

Johnstone, M. (2005). *I Had a Black Dog: His Name was Depression.* Constable & Robinson Ltd.: London, UK.

Kanter, J.W., Busch, A.M., Weeks, C.E. and Landes, S.J. (2008). The nature of clinical depression: Symptoms, syndromes, and behavior analysis. *Association for Behavioral Analysis International.* 31(1), 1–21.

Karp, D. (1996). *Speaking of Sadness: Depression, Disconnection and the Meaning of Illness.* Oxford University Press: Oxford, UK.

Katon, W., Rutter, C., Ludman, E.J., von Korff, M., Lin, E., Simon, G. et al. (2001). A randomized trial of relapse prevention of depression in primary care. *JAMA Psychiatry.* 58(3), 241–247.

Katz, D. and McHomey, C. (2002). The relationship between insomnia and health-related quality of life in patients with chronic illness. *Journal of Family Practice.* 51, 229–235.

Kelly, R. (2014). *Black Rainbow: How Words Healed Me – My Journey through Depression.* Hodder & Stoughton: London, UK.

Kembe, K. (2013). Talking with Mike Bush. http://talkingaboutsuicide.com, accessed 16 April, 2015.

Kennedy, S.H., Lam, R., Nutt, D.J. and Thase, M.E. (2004). *Treating Depression Effectively. Applying Clinical Guidelines* (2nd ed.). CRC Press: Boca Raton, FL.

Kesey, K. (1962). *One Flew over the Cuckoo's Nest.* Penguin Books: London, UK.

Kikuchi, T., Suzuki, T., Uchida, H., Watanabe, K. and Mimura, M. (2012). Coping strategies for antidepressant side effects: An Internet survey. *Journal of Affective Disorders.* 143(1–3), 89–94.

Kinsella, P. and Garland, A. (2008). *Cognitive Behavioural Therapy for Mental Health Workers: A Beginner's Guide.* Routledge: London, UK.

Kipping, C. (2013). The person with co-existing mental illness and substance use problems ('dual diagnosis'). In I. Norman and I. Ryrie (Eds.). *The Art and Science of Mental Health Nursing: Principles and Practice* (3rd ed., pp. 601–621). McGraw-Hill Education: Berkshire, England.

Klein, M.J. and Elliott, R. (2006). Client accounts of personal change in process–experiential psychotherapy: A methodologically pluralistic approach. *Psychotherapy Research.* 16(1), 91–105.

Klonsky, D., Oltmans, T. and Turkheimer, E. (2003). Deliberate self-harm in a nonclinical population: Prevalence and psychological correlates. *The American Journal of Psychiatry.* 160(8), 1501–1508.

Kokanovic, R., Bendelow, G. and Philip, B. (2013). Depression: The ambivalence of diagnosis. *Sociology of Health & Illness.* 35(3), 377–390.

Lakeman, R. and Fitzgerald, M. (2008). How people live with or get over being suicidal: A review of qualitative studies. *Journal of Advanced Nursing.* 64(2), 114–126.

Landrum, P., Beck, C., Rawlins, R. and Williams, S. (1993). In R. Rawlins, S. Williams and C. Beck (Eds.), *Mental Health – Psychiatric Nursing: A Holistic Life-Cycle Approach* (3rd ed., pp. 17–39). Mosby Year Book: London, UK.

Langbehn, D.R. and Pfohl, B. (1993). Clinical correlates of self-mutilation among psychiatric inpatients. *Annals of Clinical Psychiatry.* 5, 45–51.

Lee, L. (2007). *Living with an Impostor.* Trafford Publishing: Bloomington, IN.

Lewis, G. (2006). *Sunbathing in the Rain: A Cheerful Book about Depression.* Harper Collins Publishers: London, UK.

Lott, T. (1996). *The Scent of Dried Roses.* Viking: London, UK.

Madge, N., Hawton, K., McMahon, E., Corcoran, P., De Leo, D., Jan de Wilde, E. et al. (2011). Psychological characteristics, stressful life events and deliberate self-harm: Findings from the Child & Adolescent Self-harm in Europe (CASE) Study. *European Child & Adolescent Psychiatry.* 20(10), 499–508.

Madhukar, H. and Trivedi, M. (2004). The link between depression and physical symptoms. *Primary Care Companion to the Journal of Clinical Psychiatry.* 6(1), 12–16.

Mark, T.L., Joish, V.N., Hay, J.W., Sheehan, D., Choi, J.C., Johnston, S. and Cao, Z. (May 2009). Unintended consequences of current antidepressant use in a geriatric population: The burden of side-effects on adherence and costs. Paper presented at the *ISPOR 14th Annual International Meeting*, Orlando, FL.

Mayo Clinic (2014). What does it mean to have a nervous breakdown? http://www.mayoclinic.org, accessed 17 May, 2015.

Maytree. (2015). Maytree: A sanctuary for the suicidal. http://www.maytree.org.uk/, accessed 16 April, 2015.

Mehlum, L. (2000). The internet, suicide, and suicide prevention. *The Journal of Crisis Intervention and Suicide Prevention.* 21(4), 186–188.

Mendelsohn, C. (2012). Smoking and depression: A review. *Australian Family Physician.* 41(5), 304–307.

Mental Health Foundation (2015). Stigma and discrimination. http://www.mentalhealth.org.uk/, accessed 19 June, 2015.

Mind (2003). *The Hidden Costs of Mental Health*. Mind: London, UK.

Mind (2012). Understanding depression. www.mind.org, accessed 7 September, 2015.

Mind (2013a). About ECT. http://www.mind.org.uk/, accessed 7 September, 2015.

Mind (2013b). Making sense of art therapies. http://www.mind.org.uk, accessed 7 September, 2015.

Mittal, V., Brown, W.A. and Shorter, E. (2009). Are patients with depression at heightened risk of suicide as they begin to recover? *Psychiatric Services.* 60(3), 384–386.

Mood Café (2015). Recovery and resilience. Retrieved from http://www.moodcafe.co.uk.

Morawetz, D. (2003). Insomnia and depression: Which comes first? *Sleep Research Online.* 5(2), 77–81.

Mulligan, H. (2014). What does depression feel like? http://www.mind.org.uk/, accessed 1 July, 2015.

NAMI (2015). Depression. https://www.nami.org, accessed 20 September, 2015.

Navarro, V. (2010). Improving medication compliance in patients with depression: Use of orodispersible tablets. *Advances in Therapy.* 27(11), 785–795.

NHS Choices (2014). Depression: Trisha's story. http://www.nhs.uk, accessed 10 September, 2015.

NICE (2009). CG90: Depression in adults: The treatment and management of depression in adults. www.nice.org.uk, accessed 16 April, 2015.

NICE (2015). Depression overview. http://pathways.nice.org.uk, accessed 18 October 2015.

Nutt, D., Wilson, S. and Paterson, L. (2008). Sleep disorders as core symptoms of depression. *Dialogues in Clinical Neuroscience.* 10(3), 329–336.

Oliffe, J., Ogrodniczuk, J.S. and Han, C. (October 2010). Suicide from the perspectives of older men who experience depression. Paper presented at *ISMH World Congress 2010*, Nice, France.

Oliffe, J.L., Ogrodniczuk, J.S., Bottorff, J.L., Johnson, J.L. and Hoyak, K. (2012). "You feel like you can't live anymore": Suicide from the perspectives of Canadian men who experience depression. *Social Science and Medicine.* 74(4), 506–514.

ONS (2004). Mental health of children and young people in Great Britain, 2004. www.ons.gov.uk, accessed 12 April, 2015.

ONS (2013). Measuring national well-being – Health, 2013. www.ons.gov.uk, accessed 16 May, 2015.

ONS (2015). Statistical update on suicide. www.ons.gov.uk, accessed 16 May, 2015.

Oxford English Dictionary (2015). Stigma. http://www.oed.com, accessed 18 October, 2015.

Pampallona, S. (2004). Combined pharmacotherapy and psychological treatment for depression: A systematic review. *Archives of General Psychiatry*. 61(7), 714–719.

Papyrus. (2015). Prevention of young suicide. https://www.papyrus-uk.org/, accessed 16 April, 2015.

Parikh, S.V. and Huniewicz, P. (2015). E-health: An overview of the uses of the Internet, social media, apps, and websites for mood disorders. *Current Opinion in Psychiatry*. 28(1), 13–17.

Patient. (2015). Discussion forums. www.patient.co.uk, accessed 3 July, 2015.

Piggott, S. (2011). Let's talk about depression! http://letstalkaboutdepression.blogspot. co.uk.

Plath, S. (1963). *The Bell Jar*. Faber & Faber: London, UK.

Price, J., Cole, V. and Goodwin, G.M. (2009). Emotional side-effects of selective serotonin reuptake inhibitors: Qualitative study. *The British Journal of Psychiatry*. 195, 211–217.

Raymond, J. and Depaulo, M. (2002). *Understanding Depression: What We Know and What You Can Do About It*. John Wiley & Sons Inc.: New York.

Reekum, V., Stuss, D.T. and Ostrander, L. (2005). Apathy: Why care? *Journal of Neuropsychiatry and Clinical Neuroscience*. 17(1), 7–19.

Rice-Oxley, M. (2012). *Underneath the Lemon Tree: A Memoir of Depression and Recovery*. Little Brown: London, UK.

Royal College of Psychiatrists (2015a). Depression. http://www.rcpsych.ac.uk, accessed 3 July, 2015.

Royal College of Psychiatrists (2015b). Antidepressants. http://www.rcpsych.ac.uk, accessed 3 July, 2015.

Royal College of Psychiatrists (2015c). Information about ECT. http://www.rcpsych. ac.uk, accessed 5 July, 2015.

Samaritans. (2015). Suicide Statistics Report 2015. www.samaritans.org, accessed 30 July, 2015.

Samaritans. (2015). How we can help you. www.samaritans.org, accessed 30 July, 2015.

Selfharm UK. (2015). Discussion forum. http://selfharm.co.uk, accessed 30 July, 2015.

Serani, D. (2011). *Living with Depression: Why Biology and Biography Matter along the Path to Hope and Healing*. Rowman & Littlefield Publishers: Plymouth, England.

Sewell, A. (2007). Mine to keep. In N. Carver, J. Morrison, N. Clibbens and T. Simpson (Eds.), *Greater Goings On … (Than You Would Ever Guess …)* (p. 26). Asylum Publishing: Sheffield, England.

Shapiro, B. (2003). Building bridges between body and mind: The analysis of an adolescent with paralyzing chronic pain. *International Journal of Psychoanalysis*. 84(3), 547–561.

Smith, B. (2013). Depression and Motivation. *Phenomenology and Cognitive Sciences* 12(4), 615–635.

Smith, T.J. (2009). Clients' experience of effective psychoanalytic–psychodynamic psychotherapy for major depression: An empirical phenomenological study. Doctoral dissertation. Duquesne University: Pittsburgh, PA.

Solomon, A. (2002). *The Noonday Demon: An Anatomy of Depression*. Vintage: London, UK.

Solomon, A. (2013). Depression the secret we share. http://www.ted.com, accessed 9 June, 2015.

Stone, K. (2007). Profoundly alone. http://www.postpartumprogress.com.

Styron, W. (1990). *Darkness Visible: A Memoir of Madness*. Vintage: London, UK.

Sullivan, L.E., Fiellin, D.A. and O'Connor, P.G. (2005). The prevalence and impact of alcohol problems in major depression: A systematic review. *The American Journal of Medicine*. 118(4), 330–341.

Survivors of Suicide (2014). Suicide Frequently Asked Questions. http://www.survivorsofsuicide.com, accessed 16 April, 2015.

The Site. (2015). Discussion forum. www.thesite.org, accessed 30 July, 2015.

Time to Change. (2015). Blogs. http://www.time-to-change.org.uk, accessed 26 August, 2015.

Time to Change (2012). Personal narrative. http://www.time-to-change.org.uk, accessed 5 April, 2015.

Time to Change (2014a). Personal narrative. http://www.time-to-change.org.uk, accessed 8 April, 2015.

Time to Change (2014b). Personal narrative. http://www.time-to-change.org.uk, accessed 5 April, 2015.

Time to Change (2014c). Personal narrative. http://www.time-to-change.org.uk, accessed 6 April, 2015.

Time to Change (2015). Personal narrative. http://www.time-to-change.org.uk, accessed 5 April, 2015.

Townend, E., Tinson, D., Kwan, J. and Sharpe, M. (2010). 'Feeling sad and useless': An investigation into personal acceptance of disability and its association with depression following stroke. *Clinical Rehabilitation*. 24(6), 555–564.

Trescothick, M. (2008). *Coming Back to Me*. HarperCollins: London, UK.

Van Lith, T., Fenner, P. and Schofield, M. (2011). The lived experience of art making as a companion to the mental health recovery process. *Disability and Rehabilitation*. 33(8), 652–660.

Vatne, M. and Naden, D. (2012). Finally, it became too much – Experiences and reflections in the aftermath of attempted suicide. *Scandinavian Journal of Caring Sciences*. 26(2), 304–312.

Vicarious Therapy (2010). ECT. http://vicarioustherapy.blogspot.co.uk, accessed 30 July, 2015.

Vincent, R. (2007). Early closing Thursday. In N. Carver, J. Morrison, N. Clibbens, and T. Simpson (Eds.), *Greater Goings On … (Than You Would Ever Guess …)* (p. 43). Asylum Publishing: Sheffield, England.

Weisz, J.R., McCarty, C.A. and Valeri, S.M. (2006). Effects of psychotherapy for depression in children and adolescents: A meta-analysis. *Psychological Bulletin*. 132(1), 132–149.

Welch, D. (2010). *Pulling Myself Together*. Sidgwick & Jackson: London, UK.

WHO (2012). Depression stats. http://www.who.int, accessed 27 May, 2015.

WHO (2014). WHO Mental Health Gap Action Programme. http://www.who.int, accessed 27 May, 2015.

Widemalm, M. and Hjarthag, F. (2015). The forum as a friend: Parental mental illness and communication on open internet forums. *Social Psychiatry and Psychiatric Epidemiology*. 22, 1–7.

Williams, C. (2006). *Overcoming Depression and Low Mood: A Five Areas Approach* (2nd ed.). Hodder Arnold: London, UK.

Williams, J.M.G., Healy, D., Teasdale, J.D., White, W. and Paykel, E.S. (1990). Dysfunctional attitudes and vulnerability to persistent depression. *Psychological Medicine*. 20, 375–381.

Williams, M., Teasdale, J., Segal, Z. and Kabat-Zinn, J. (2007). *The Mindful Way through Depression: Freeing Yourself from Chronic Unhappiness*. Guilford Press: New York.

Williams, M.R. (2012). *Depression and Bipolar Disorder: Your Guide to Recovery*. Bull: Lancaster, England.

Winnicott, D.W. (1962). Ego integration in child development. In D.W. Winnicott (Ed.), *The Maturational Processes and the Facilitating Environment* (pp. 56–63). Hogarth Press: London, UK.

Winnicott, D.W. (1964). Psychosomatic disorder. In C. Winnicott, R. Shepherd and M. Davis (Eds.), *Psychoanalytic Explorations* (1989) (pp. 103–118). Harvard University Press: Cambridge, UK.

Woodgate, R.L. (2006). Living in the shadow of fear: Adolescents' lived experience of depression. *Journal of Advanced Nursing*. 56(3), 261–269.

Wurtzel, E. (1994). *Prozac Nation*. Quartet Books: London, UK.

Yalom, I. (2005). *Theory and Practice of Group Psychotherapy* (5th ed.). Basic Books: New York.

Yap, M.B., Reayley, N.J. and Jorm, A.F. (2013). Associations between stigma and help-seeking intentions and beliefs: Findings from an Australian national survey of young people. *Psychiatry Research*. 210(3), 1154–1160.

'My brain won't slow down'
Living with extremes of mood

INTRODUCTION

This chapter is concerned with the experience of living with extreme mood states at both ends of the spectrum, depressed and elevated. Whilst many of the features experienced with lowered mood might seem similar to those already addressed in Chapter 4, there are distinct differences for people given the very sharp contrast between these polarised opposites. Having experienced, for example, periods of euphoria, high productivity and a sense of heightened awareness, there will be a keen awareness of what is subsequently different or lost when mood significantly lowers. The experiences covered in this chapter relate to what is diagnostically categorised as bipolar disorder, a condition formally called 'manic depression'. The term 'bipolar disorder' is unpopular though with many service users who prefer the term 'bipolar' regarding their condition more as an illness as opposed to a disorder (RCP, 2012). Therefore, it is this shortened term which will mainly be used in this chapter.

WHAT IS BIPOLAR?

Bipolar is a severe mental health condition characterised by significant mood swings lasting for weeks or months and includes manic highs and depressive lows (see Figure 5.1). The majority of individuals affected experience alternating episodes of mania and depression (see Box 5.1) although between episodes may have long periods of stable functioning. Low or depressive states may be accompanied with feelings of intense depression and despair, whilst high or manic states are characterised by feelings of extreme happiness and elation. There are also mixed states experienced by some with depressed mood. Both males and females of any age and from any social or ethnic background are affected and it can occur when work, study, family or emotional pressures are at their greatest. In women it can also be triggered by childbirth or during the menopause. Management of the illness is normally through strategies involving medication, health care, therapy and self-management (RCP, 2012).

- One to two percent of the population experiences a lifetime prevalence of bipolar.
- The impact and devastation of bipolar extends to parents and partners.
- The World Health Organisation has identified bipolar as one of the top causes of lost years of life and health in 15–44 year olds, ranking above war, violence and schizophrenia.
- It takes an average of 10.5 years to receive a correct diagnosis for bipolar in the United Kingdom.
- Bipolar increases the risk of suicide by up to 20 times.
- People with bipolar spend around 50% of their lives after onset with significant symptoms, mainly depression.
- Treatment of bipolar is still hampered by misunderstanding and severe stigma.
- Bipolar impacts every aspect of one's life especially relationships, work and day-to-day living.

Figure 5.1 Bipolar – the facts. (From Bipolar UK, Information, 2015, http://www.bipolaruk.org.uk, accessed 12 July, 2015; RCP, Bipolar, 2012, http://www.rcpsych.ac.uk, accessed 12 July, 2015.)

TYPES

BIPOLAR I

This type is recognised when there has been at least one manic episode which lasted for more than 1 week. Some people with bipolar I will have only manic episodes, although most will also have periods of depression.

BIPOLAR II

The type here is affirmed where there has been more than one episode of severe depression, but only mild manic episodes ('hypomania'). With this type, depressive episodes can be more frequent and are more intensely experienced than hypomanic episodes. Bipolar II can remain under-diagnosed with hypomanic behaviour presenting as high-functioning behaviour. Of particular concern amongst the bipolar spectra is the elevated risk of suicide amongst those with bipolar II.

RAPID CYCLING

This type is identified when more than four mood swings have occurred within a 12-month period. It affects between 10% and 20% of people with bipolar and can happen with both types I and II.

CYCLOTHYMIA

The mood swings seen here are generally not as severe as those in full bipolar but can be longer. This can develop into full bipolar (Bipolar UK, 2015; RCP, 2012).

Box 5.1 The experience of bipolar

Life is....

a teetering

between the two[a]

on a virtual tightrope

with Heaven above

and Hell below;

seeing always

the seething pit

and the summoning

stars.

Knowing the pendulum of your

Moods,

You fear

The fall into Hell

And the flight to the

Gods

In equal measure:

Put one foot wrong

And you're gone.

So you stand and stare,

Transfixed, and scared

To move

Alone.

Source: Eden, G., Manic depression, in: Carver, N. et al., eds., *Greater Goings On …* *(Than You Would Ever Guess …)*, Asylum Publishing, Sheffield, England, 2007, p. 35.
[a] Mania and depression.

BIPOLAR: 'THE CELEBRITY'S CONDITION'?

There have been many people in the public eye over recent years who have reportedly experienced bipolar, leading this condition to be informally regarded as a 'celebrity's affliction'. Whilst arguments can be levelled towards some people for 'jumping on the bandwagon' or trivialising what is a serious and distressing condition, it is evident that a large number of celebrities (and non-celebrities) are indeed living with bipolar. People in the public eye who experience bipolar provide important role models helping to challenge some of the stigmatising beliefs associated with mental health problems. Here, for example, are likeable and respected icons (Stephen Fry and Frank Bruno), individuals who have shown periods of great productivity and entertained or impressed us with the quality of their work. Such periods though are generally connected with elevated mood

Adam Ant (singer – Adam and the Ants)

Russell Brand (comedian)

Frank Bruno (boxer)

Ray Davies (musician – The Kinks)

Richard Dreyfuss (actor)

Carrie Fisher (actor)

Stephen Fry (comedian/TV presenter)

Mel Gibson (actor)

Terry Hall (singer – The Specials)

Kerry Katona (musician – Atomic Kitten)

Vivien Leigh (actor)

Spike Milligan (comedian)

Graham Obree (cyclist)

Bill Oddie (comedian/TV presenter)

Axl Rose Hall (singer – Guns N' Roses)

Nina Simone (singer)

Tony Slattery (comedian/TV presenter)

David Walliams (comedian/writer)

Ruby Wax (comedian/TV presenter)

Robbie Williams (singer)

Brian Wilson (musician – The Beach Boys)

Catherine Zeta-Jones (actress)

What are your thoughts about this list?

Figure 5.2 Celebrities with bipolar.

states and can be contrasted by periods of inactivity when mood is depressed. A list of celebrities who have experienced bipolar is included in Figure 5.2.

SECTION 1: EXPERIENCING BIPOLAR

First experience

Interview narratives

To me at first I just felt slightly elated and I thought that was normal after giving birth and being happy. But it was other people, especially my husband who began to pick up on things. My speech became faster and a bit pressured and in conversations I would jump from one subject to another and he was finding it difficult to follow.

It has made it difficult to concentrate, even something like trying to follow a TV programme or read a book.

I would start with one conversation and then flip to something else ... other people were picking up on that.

> My brain won't slow down.
>
> [When depressed] I lose my appetite. I find it hard to sleep, I lose my motivation. I don't really enjoy doing things. I don't like seeing a lot of people and hide away.
>
> I just felt so miserable that I just wanted to go to sleep and stay asleep.

The initial experiences with bipolar can be confusing and bewildering, especially given the prolonged amount of time from first symptoms to diagnosis which can average 13 years (Bipolar UK, 2015). The first signs that something might be wrong can be connected with elevated or lowered mood states or a combination of both. Rachel, a 15-year-old girl who had experienced episodes of depression in the past, began talking very quickly and appeared to have excess energy. She went through a period of barely sleeping or eating, saying things that did not make sense to others such as her being a Taiwanese princess. Whilst many behaviours appeared out of character for her such as swearing and being flirtatious, she told others:

I've never felt so great – I'm flying. I'm eleven on a scale of one to ten.

Bailey and Shooter (2009)

A diagnosis of bipolar was subsequently confirmed. Initial symptoms can progress at different rates and for some deterioration in functioning can be very rapid. As Jamison (1995, p. 36) recounts:

I lost my mind rather rapidly. At first everything seemed so easy. I raced about like a crazed weasel, bubbling with plans and enthusiasms, immersed in sports, and staying up all night, night after night, out with friends, reading everything that wasn't nailed down, filling manuscript books with poems and fragments of plays … I felt great. Not just great, I felt really great.

As she recounts she did finally stop, coming to a grinding halt. The quality of the experiences narrated here illustrates signs of elation and vibrancy. There is a sense of feeling fantastic or 'on top of the world', filled with productivity and enthusiasm. This is very different to symptoms felt at the depressive end of the spectrum, as, for example, Johnston's (2002, p. 43) which felt oppressive and menacing:

This depression was sneaky and insidious, gradually working its way into all facets of my life, gradually removing every bastion of self-worth and self-confidence that I had.

It will evidently be more noticeable here that something is wrong and that help is needed. For those experiencing an elevation of mood it might only be when others notice or when one's mood drops that support is sought. This can be difficult though owing to fears around stigma and critical responses from others. Effective health promotion and education around the condition helps by lessening the trepidation amongst those seeking help. The storyline featuring Stacey Slater being diagnosed as bipolar in the television soap *Eastenders* was extremely impactful. Following this the Bipolar Disorder Research Network (BDRN) received a record number of visitors to their website and the number of young people calling helplines more than doubled (BBC, 2010). This shows the importance of creating greater awareness and acceptability through relating the condition of bipolar to people who are in a sense *known* and where the experience can be better contextualised and understood.

DIAGNOSIS

> What do you feel a person's feelings might be on receipt of a bipolar diagnosis?

The receipt of a bipolar diagnosis is likely to evoke very strong emotions including relief and hope as well as fear and distress. Each person will have their own sense as to what this diagnostic term means to them. Feelings such as bewilderment, fear and uncertainty are all evidenced in narratives on the Bipolar UK website through the discussion theme *newly diagnosed and overwhelmed*. A number of postings here are from individuals asking for advice and help around self-managing without medication, recognising warning signs, coping with erratic behaviour such as overspending and hypersexuality, depressive episodes and irritability. A key message emerging from discussion threads demonstrates that having a diagnosis can provide a helpful point of reference for those diagnosed, their families and friends. It is a point at which people clearly have many questions which need asking as well as a significant need for support and reassurance. This site importantly provides a valuable starting place for receiving understanding, acceptance and help. The feeling of relief on receiving a diagnosis is also reflected in narratives located elsewhere. Christina, a young person with bipolar recounts:

> Once I was diagnosed as bipolar I was able to understand and come to terms with my illness.
>
> Bailey and Shooter (2009)

Her experience perhaps is not representative of the majority of adolescents for whom the application of the diagnostic process can be complex and stressful. Yeloglu et al. (2011) reflect that bipolar can occur with different clinical manifestations in the adolescent stage compared to the adult form and usually results in a wrong diagnosis. This is supported by Bowden's (2009) study which found people with bipolar being subject to high rates of misdiagnosis. This was explained in part through individuals seeking help for depressive episodes and not recognising or reporting manic or hypomanic symptomatology.

If correctly applied having a diagnosis can be helpful in having a means of conceptualising and making sense of what one has been struggling with the following:

> Suddenly the solar system snaps into place, and at the centre is this sun; I have a word. Bipolar. Now it will be better. Now it has a name, and if it has a name, it's a real thing, not merely my imagination gone wild. If it has a name, if it isn't

merely an utter failure on my part, if it's a disease, bipolar disorder, then it has an answer. Then it has a cure.

Hornbacher (2008, p. 67)

This narrative highlights a sense of hope. There is a reason here to explain what she has been experiencing coupled with corresponding treatments and interventions. Whilst a diagnosis can bring hope and clarity, it is also worth bearing in mind other people's experiences which may be less positive or hopeful. One particular issue concerns the feeling of being labelled with a 'mental health' condition and the stigmatising, fearful connotations connected with it. In Johnston's (2002, p. 10) case, her diagnosis was met with a position of denial:

These doctors and nurses were kidding themselves that I had manic depression. It was all lies.

The initial sense of shock can evidently provoke self-protecting responses which are instinctively engaged. It is evidently difficult to reconcile oneself to a position of acceptance with the possession of a mental health condition. The feelings around one's diagnosis are not necessarily a fixed state with emotions liable to vary:

So how does it feel to have finally been diagnosed with bipolar disorder? Initially I was punching the air … Then the reality set in. The realisation of the implications, for my life, my work, my driving license even, what I would have to or not have to disclose to employers, to friends, to family. My moods would shift from elation to despair in a matter of minutes.

Time to Change (2014a)

This highlights the needs for healthcare professionals to be alert to the changing feelings and thoughts of service users concerning their diagnosis and to support them accordingly.

TELLING PEOPLE

Confiding in others about one's diagnosis of bipolar and experienced problems appears to evoke very mixed reactions. A commonly held concern is of being dismissed, ridiculed or stigmatised. Whilst some narratives relate a lack of understanding and poor support received others highlight the invaluable help and acceptance they have been given. Positive experiences apply especially when telling family members or peers – other people with bipolar. Friends and work colleagues seem less predictable and prone to react in different ways dependent upon the nature of the relationship established with them or their ability and desire to comprehend the meaning of someone else's difficulties.

A blogger relates the insensitive treatment she received from her friends

who didn't understand what had happened. They posted statuses on Facebook about me and told people on the course that I was 'a psycho' and 'crazy'. This caused me to feel isolated and alone.

Time to Change (2014b)

The intention of these 'friends' is hard comprehend and certainly shows a marked lack of understanding about this condition or any sensitivity towards Cara. Responses such as these reinforce concerns people hold about opening up to others and can have a very debilitating effect. The workplace can be a particularly difficult arena to confide in others because of worries about potential consequences. Another Time to Change (2014c) blogger sums up her initial thoughts when contemplating telling people:

> When the time came to meet with my boss, I felt both frightened and ashamed. I didn't want her to look at me 'like that' … I had to say the words 'I'm bipolar'. I hated the way they felt in my mouth. I hated the space they took up in the air, as though the words were taunting me. But most of all, I hated becoming that employee, with that problem.

The impact that a mental health diagnosis can have upon a person's perceptions of self in relation to others is very strongly expressed here. The stigma often associated with mental health problems can become internalised with those 'labelled' feeling somewhat different and inferior to others who by comparison are perceived as 'normal'. What is important to note here is the *perception* of how one feels and the subsequent impact this has upon a person. One blogger received a less than favourable response from her boss but fortunately her colleagues were much more supportive:

> I started by telling a few colleagues at work who I have also formed a friendship with and was overwhelmed by their response. They are trying to understand the condition and are being so supportive.
>
> Time to Change (2012a)

Perhaps one of the most important elements here concerns the statement 'they are trying to understand'. Whilst a number of misconceptions may still need correcting, what matters is the intention and desire amongst others to grasp meaning around one's mental health experience. Increased awareness and understanding around bipolar helps to change attitudes and encourage more supportive responses. It appears from various narratives that negative reactions are largely influenced through lack of knowledge about what the realities of living with bipolar are. This supports the work of campaigning groups such as Time to Change who challenge attitudes through sharing stories of actual experience.

LOWERED MOOD

Everyone experiences lowered moods from time to time although within clinical depression or bipolar the feelings are of an acute nature, impacting significantly upon a person's ability to function. Maczka et al.'s (2010) study found consensus between service users and psychiatrists in that depression is the most burdensome episode in the course of bipolar. Figure 5.3 illustrates some of the ways in which a person will experience depression.

A major difficulty for those who are depressed concerns the lack of motivation, energy or drive to effect any change. This is illustrated by Marya Hornbacher (2008, p. 132) who states:

If you become depressed, you will notice some of these changes:

Emotional
- Feelings of unhappiness that don't go away
- Feeling that you want to burst into tears for no reason
- Losing interest in things
- Being unable to enjoy things
- Feeling restless and agitated
- Losing self-confidence
- Feeling useless, inadequate and hopeless
- Feeling more irritable than usual
- Thinking of suicide

Thinking
- Can't think positively or hopefully
- Finding it hard to make even simple decisions
- Difficulty in concentrating

Physical
- Losing appetite and weight
- Difficulty in getting to sleep
- Waking earlier than usual
- Feeling utterly tired
- Constipation
- Going off sex

Behaviour
- Difficulty in starting or completing things – even everyday chores
- Crying a lot – or feeling like you want to cry, but not being able to
- Avoiding contact with other people

Figure 5.3 Depression. (From RCP, Bipolar, 2012, http://www.rcpsych.ac.uk, accessed 12 July, 2015.)

I do not have the energy to pull myself free. I do not have the energy to even care that I am trapped. This is beyond caring, beyond a will to die. Death is there but you can barely lift your hand to reach out to it, and you cringe at the faintest suggestion of light … I am underwater. I am a body. I follow the world through my telescope. I am drugged, and so feel nothing at all.

This personal reflection alludes to a number of sensations including powerlessness and helplessness. It also highlights the sense of feeling trapped, unable to move or affect any change. There is a strong experience of detachment and distancing from both her emotions and the world around her. Acknowledging this experience, it is understandable that a person can feel very strongly if told, for example, by others to 'pull yourself together'. This type of response fails to acknowledge the depth and intensity of a person's felt and lived experience.

A depressive phase can also be characterised by a sense of numbness, self-preoccupation and closure concerning external stimuli. This can be highlighted through the process of 're-awakening' which can take place when emerging from a depressive episode. As expressed by Stuart Goddard (2006, p. 322), better known as the singer Adam Ant:

> Gradually as time passed, my medication was modified and I came out of the deepest part of the depression and more aware of my circumstances. … Eventually as I progressed I was allowed a whole day out. On those days we would go for walks, and I could feel the cool breeze and fresh air on my face, which was what I needed to wake me up. For the first time in a long while I could see everyday life passing by and hear the sounds of the streets.

This narrative distinctly expresses the sensation of re-awakening or re-emerging into the world indicating a significant shift of awareness and appreciation of fine detail. The loss of this fine detail when one's mood becomes depressed is likely to be felt very keenly by those who have also experienced elevated mood states. A number of personal narratives commenting upon elevated mood reflect upon the nuances that can be heard in a piece of music, the exquisite and varied tastes enjoyed in a food item or the dazzling colours and construction glimpsed within a painting. This clearly illustrates a significant shift from the depressed state where these same items cannot be enjoyed, appreciated or even noticed providing a real sense of loss.

ELEVATED MOOD

Elevated mood can incorporate a sense of well-being, energy and optimism or what Tricia Thorpe calls her 'giddy behaviour' (Your Voices, 2012). Feeling euphoric or high can indeed represent states which are desired or sought after. The intensity or duration of such feelings though can be very detrimental, affecting a person's thinking and judgement. Individuals are prone to behaving in embarrassing, socially inappropriate or even dangerous ways. Day-to-day life can be severely affected with relationships, work and study significantly impacted upon. There can be severe financial implications with excessive spending engaged in. The range of issues present with elevated mood or mania can be seen in Figure 5.4.

Kay Jamison (1995, p. 79) expresses very vividly the heightened sense of perception present when her mood was elevated:

> My awareness and experience of sounds in general were intense. Individual notes from a horn, an oboe, or a cello became exquisitely poignant. I heard each note alone, all notes together, and then each and all with piercing beauty and clarity.

This is clearly in sharp contrast to the experiences related earlier during a depressive episode. It illustrates a phase where individuals can strongly feel alive and vibrant. It is an experience which many people are desirous of maintaining and prolonging and can cause despair when feeling one's heightened mood gradually eroding. Attempts to maintain this state include self-medicating through drink and drugs or avoiding sleep, all of which later have detrimental effects.

If you become manic, you may notice that you are experience the following:

Emotional
- Very happy and excited
- Irritated with other people who don't share your optimistic outlook
- Feeling more important than usual

Thinking
- Full of new and exciting ideas
- Moving quickly from one idea to another
- Hearing voices that other people can't hear

Physical
- Full of energy
- Unable or unwilling to sleep
- More interested in sex

Behaviour
- Making plans that are grandiose and unrealistic
- Very active, moving around very quickly
- Behaving unusually
- Talking very quickly – other people may find it hard to understand what you are talking about
- Making odd decisions on the spur of the moment, sometimes with disastrous consequences
- Recklessly spending your money
- Overfamiliar or recklessly critical with other people
- Less inhibited in general

Figure 5.4 Mania. (From RCP, Bipolar, 2012, http://www.rcpsych.ac.uk, accessed 12 July, 2015.)

The speed at which a person feels they are operating can pose difficulties:

I knew I was insane, my thoughts were so fast that I couldn't remember the beginning of a sentence halfway through. Fragments of ideas, images, sentences raced around and around in my mind … I wanted desperately to slow down but could not.

Jamison (1995, p. 82)

It can make it hard to concentrate or attend to things but at times can also feel exhilarating. This is reflected by Carrie Fisher (Wilson, 2006):

When you're galloping along at great speed it's better than any drug you could take … you're just so enthusiastic about everyone and everyone must be enthusiastic about you.

She went on though to relate the problems of going faster than others who were unable to keep up with her and the problem this poses for both parties. The person with elevated mood is likely to feel annoyed and frustrated with those who are not in synch with them whilst others are left feeling bewildered and confused by the rapidity of the person's thoughts and speech. This can be seen with Michelle's Story (DBSA, 2015) where she relates to having

> an unending supply of ideas for books and screenplays I wanted to write. I was making staggering realizations about the secrets of life. But I was also having more and more problems getting my point across to other people or carrying on any type of logical conversation at all. When no one understood my ideas and revelations, I became suspicious and paranoid.

The speed and nature of thoughts that accompany this elevated mood state can also be matched by periods of intense productivity. There are many examples of this with gifted and creative individuals, for example, Virginia Woolf (1953, p. 74), who was thought to have had bipolar, wrote:

> One thing, in considering my state of mind now, seems to me beyond dispute; that I have at last, bored down into my oil well, and can't scribble fast enough to bring it all to the surface … I have never felt this rush and urgency before.

Similar experiences are also reported with the comedian Spike Milligan and the composer Robert Schumann who had intense periods of productivity followed by periods of inertia (Morris, 2006).

Another behavioural manifestation includes excessive spending and Cheney (2008) recounts a shopping spree in which her entire savings were used up. It included buying whatever took her fancy and involved many items of which she clearly had no use. Stephen Fry (Wilson, 2006) illustrated some of the dynamics involved here when out shopping accompanied by a psychotherapist. He recounted finding it hard to stop buying items, many of which he had no real need for and reflected that spending was rewarding, helping him feel alive. He likened this process to a hunt with the joy (and necessity) of the kill. There is though a corresponding *crash* which is experienced later along with feelings of guilt and a sense of squalor.

> How might a person feel within each mood state given the sharp contrast between them?

Suicidal ideation

Bipolar increases a person's mortality rate with both natural causes and 'unnatural' causes such as suicide and risky behaviours being key contributors (Ketter, 2010). This is borne out by Thangavelu et al.'s (2012) study which found that those with bipolar have a higher risk of committing suicide than the general population and noted that poor impulse control is likely to be a contributory factor. Song et al. (2012) examined risk factors for suicide amongst those with bipolar and identified a number of strong predictors including younger age at onset, lifetime history of auditory hallucinations and history of antidepressant use. Antecedent depressive episodes and psychotic symptoms predicted the first suicide attempt in patients with bipolar. Finseth et al.'s (2012) study identified suicidal risk factors as a predominant depressive course of illness and a comorbid alcohol and substance use. The desire to take one's own life when plagued by despairing or chaotic thoughts can at times feel very compelling, as evidenced by a number of narratives. Brian Adams (2003, p. 43) recalls:

> When my heart sinks at the prospect of another day of being me, I am usually in a condition in which wherever I go I view all high fittings from the point of view of the ability to hold a rope with me at the end of it.

In a related narrative, Neil Walton (2007) expresses very eloquently cutting into his arm with a scalpel, slowly testing the pain factor and seeing how far he could go. He reflected that he might not have been around now if he had been able to locate a gun. This is similarly reflected in many other narratives which relate deliberate attempts to end one's tormented existence or careless, negligent behaviour with an ambivalent attitude to one's health or safety. The first element can be illustrated by Kay Jamison's (1995, p. 114) experience of feeling that care was not working and her resolve to kill herself as she could not stand the pain any longer:

> a pitiless, unrelenting pain that offers no window of hope.

Her resolution was such that she bought a gun, visited the eighth floor of a building and took a Lithium overdose. Fortunately she survived and recovered, helped by what she regarded to be exceptionally good support from friends, health care professionals and family. This absolute need for supportive and accepting people is also indicated by Hornbacher (2008) who was rushed to hospital after inflicting serious cuts on her arm. Therefore, health carers need to be aware of the very real risk of suicide or death through negligence and lack of caring which those with bipolar can pose.

Psychotic symptoms

If an episode of mania or depression becomes very severe, individuals may develop psychotic symptoms. These can be experienced within either polarised mood state. If elevated, for example, a person can have grandiose beliefs feeling as if they have special powers and abilities or are on an important mission. In a depressive episode, individuals can feel uniquely guilty, worse than anybody else or as if they do not exist. Hornbacher (2008, p. 118) writes about her shifting reality and dreamlike state whilst wandering through the desert in a narrative reminiscent of Malcolm Lowry's (1947) *Under the Volcano*. She expresses the sense of her external world being experienced as fragments flashing by:

> When you are mad, mad like this, you don't know it. Reality is what you see. When what you see shifts, departing from anyone else's reality, it's still reality to you.

The essence here concerns the fact this *altered reality* has become *her reality*. It illustrates the importance of acknowledging the perceptions of those concerned. If addressed from an emotional perspective her narrative is very illustrative and expressive. This shows her feeling disconnected, lost and frightened.

In bipolar, disorders of reality can include experiencing hallucinations, sensations that are not perceived by others (RCP, 2012). Katie (Mind, 2014a), who has bipolar, describes the changing nature of her voice hearing experience when experiencing different mood states:

> During mania, the voices can be comforting … They give me ideas and fill me with confidence that then elevates my mood further … The voices have become my friends and I think I would miss them if they were gone.

However, as her mood drops:

> When I'm severely depressed I have heard screaming and shouting in my head … The screaming is constant and then there is a voice shouting 'Everyone hates you', 'You're worthless' and 'Why don't you kill yourself'. It frightens me immensely.

Similarly, visual hallucinations can be experienced as menacing and scary or supportive and benign. Suzy Johnston (2002) experienced terrifying hallucinations observing the floor turn into water and a creature emerging from the wall. In contrast to this, Rod (Wilson, 2006) related seeing angels an experience he welcomed as

> when you've walked with angels all the pain and suffering is worthwhile.

An illustrative point here relates to the fact that hallucinatory experience, although fantastical or difficult to comprehend can provide an indicator of underlying mood. This provides an element with which health carers can engage with and provided needed support.

EXCESSIVE AND RISKY BEHAVIOUR

A particular difficulty for people with bipolar concerns uncontrollable excesses of behaviour or engagement in risky ventures. It relates to aspects such as hypersexuality, overspending, excessive drinking and aggressiveness. The BP Hope (2014) website includes accounts of lavish spending upon items as diverse as apartments, sporting equipment, holidays, hairstyles or linen:

> I can't tell you how many duvets I got … I could spend $1000 on napkins and candles.
>
> *bp Magazine* for Bipolar – bphope.com

Indeed, for one individual featured here the spending amounted to over $100,000 in a single year. It appears that the money imparted can be upon items or services in an attempt to help people feel better:

> I think the spending was how I coped with not coping.
>
> *bp Magazine* for Bipolar – bphope.com

It can also be influenced by states of agitation and restless as recounted by Cheney (2008, p. 164):

> Colours kept exploding behind my closed eyes. Words and numbers glowed and pulsed like neon signs … I hadn't slept in five days.

It was in this state that she felt the urge for movement, running in circles around her garden before getting in her car and driving away. She then bought 14 large kites (for her classmates) which she then 'set free' when the weather turned stormy. This whole narrative section reflects a whirlwind of restless activity where the kites were bought as a spontaneous, impulsive purchase fitting her fleeting thoughts at that moment in time. The excessive, uncontrolled spending can quickly drain a person's savings and leave them with large debts. Lakhani (2008) reports upon the debts of £35,000 accrued by PhD student Rachael Watson who was subsequently pursued relentlessly by her bank with frequent phone calls and letters demanding repayment. This stress engaged with this will further tax a person's dwindling coping resources.

Perhaps one of the most emotionally fraught aspects concerns the area of hypersexuality which can impact strongly upon individuals' thoughts and feelings. This can cause difficulties in accepting one's behaviour or forgiving oneself as well as worries about how others might respond. As Mind (2013) point out:

> You may not be aware of the changes in your attitude or behaviour while you are having a manic episode. However, after a manic phase is over, you may be shocked at what you have done and the effect that it has had.

This illustrates the need for support including opportunities to make sense of one's thoughts and feelings over what a person has been involved with. Natasha Tracy provoked a fascinating discussion around the question of accountability in her blog 'Bipolar Burble'. Her feeling is that unless psychotic, people need to take personal responsibility:

> If I do something, it was me doing it and no one else. No doubt, what I've done may be highly influenced by a disease that is not my fault, but I still committed the action and have to deal with the consequences … You can't just throw up your hands and say, 'yes, I had an affair because I was hypersexual – it wasn't my fault, it was the bipolar'. That just increases the harm that you have caused. I know it's a bitter pill to swallow and it's hard to take responsibility for things that are so influenced by bipolar, but I believe it is an important one. It's important not only for our own wellbeing but also for the wellbeing of those around us.
>
> Tracy (2014)

Responses to this were very mixed. Those in opposition felt that what was said was either categorically wrong or dependent upon the severity of a person's symptoms. A number of people though supported Tracy's statement pointing to preventative measures or lifestyle choices a person can make.

What do you feel about the differing responses noted here?

SELF-MEDICATION

A prominent means for individuals coping with fluctuating mood states has been through *treating* themselves by self-medicating. This can relate to the use of various non-prescription pharmaceutical substances and through the use of alcohol or tobacco. Studies indicate that bipolar and substance-use disorders commonly occur in the same individual with bipolar having a higher prevalence of substance-use disorders than any other psychiatric illness (Swann, 2010). The significance for those concerned relates to Swann's (2010) findings that those self-medicating have a more severe course of bipolar, including earlier onset, more frequent episodes and more complications, including anxiety and stress-related disorders, aggressive behaviour, legal problems and suicidal ideation. Bipolar and substance-use disorders share common mechanisms, including impulsivity, poor modulation of motivation and responses to rewarding stimuli and susceptibility to behavioural sensitisation.

Ward (2011) found a high incidence of substance use in the bipolar population which increases negative outcomes and changes the illness presentation. The six themes that emerged from analysis of formulated meanings were

- Life is hard
- Feeling the effects
- Trying to escape
- Spiritual support
- Being pushed beyond the limits
- A negative connotation

These aspects reflect experiences recounted within a range of autobiographical narratives and Hornbacher (2008) in particular related how alcohol helps to lift her depression, although causing it to rise rapidly into mania. This highlights the problem of increasing one's instability through the consumption of illicit substances which is reflected in Ros Morris' (2008) account of her son's problems being made worse through his use of drugs. Reasons for using drugs or alcohol are either attempts to seek respite from troubling symptoms or to try and prevent one's mood from dropping. This section can be widened to encompass other maladaptive self-coping mechanisms including lifestyle factors, dietary choices or approaches to sleep. This can especially apply when people are aware of elevated mood states beginning to lessen. The desperate need to hold onto one's state of productivity and vitality is added to through fears around progressing towards a depressive state. This can lead to unhelpful approaches being engaged with such as excess caffeine consumption or attempts to avoid sleep.

It is evident that lifestyle factors require careful attendance in order to support one's prolonged ability to cope. As illustrated by Jones et al. (2009), self-responsibility and lifestyle changes such as attending to diet, relaxation, sleep patterns, eating and exercise will add protective functions, whereas a chaotic lifestyle leaves a person more at risk of mood changes. Examples about the detrimental impact of not attending sufficiently to one's lifestyle are illustrated by Hornbacher (2008), Morris (2008) and Cheney (2008), all of whom illustrate the detrimental effects it had upon their (or family member's) health and well-being.

SECTION 2: EXPERIENCING SUPPORT

Interview narratives

He [the Dr] just sat there with a bemused look on his face and said I think you've got bipolar affective disorder, what do you think to that?

I got really quite severe side effects to one of the medications and didn't realise at first what was happening … it affected my speech because my tongue was getting so tight I couldn't talk, I couldn't lie down because then I couldn't breathe.

Some of the side effects and physical problems you get from taking the medication are worse sometimes than some of the things that you experience through the original illness.

I was assaulted [in hospital] by a female patient.

I felt bored on the ward as there wasn't enough to do. There was a tiny bit of occupational therapy but very little.

I've lost a couple of friends … I remember one saying I can't visit you in hospital, I don't like hospitals and certainly not those sorts of hospitals.

I had counselling for quite a long period which helped.

I didn't feel confident going to talk to people. She [therapist] broke it down and we looked at alternative thoughts and that helped me look at it in a different way.

We did some mindfulness as well which I found helpful.

I want to be involved in the decisions in my own care and not to just be told – this is what's happening, this is what to take, and this is what we're going to do.

For quite a while, I went to one of the bipolar support groups which is now Bipolar UK … it was very, very helpful.

This section outlines a range of interventions and the experiences of those accessing them. It includes approaches such as psychological therapies, medication, in-patient care, creative approaches, peer support and help received from family and friends.

PSYCHOLOGICAL THERAPIES

What do you think a person with bipolar might expect or want from psychotherapy?

An important intervention for those with bipolar involves psychotherapeutic work. This provides one with opportunities to process what one is experiencing and the accompanying thoughts and feelings:

I realised through talking, talking about experiencing bipolar has lifted me from the moments of absolute darkness. It has helped me to accept the weight of the diagnosis, allowed me to mentally move on from the past and taught me that there's still a lot to look forward to in my future.

Time to Change (2014d)

This recollection reflects the value in having space to talk and express oneself and to start making sense of what one is experiencing. There is also a powerful communication here about renewed hope and optimism, aspects commonly lost when struggling with distressing symptoms. Maxine (Your Stories, 2014) found talking therapies helpful in valuing herself and making sense of her mental health experience:

It was great to have someone who believed in me, it helped raise my confidence so I felt self-assured.

The feeling of acceptance from another person is crucial, validating and attending to one's distress. It is also supported by the personal qualities and degree of sensitivity shown by the therapist. This is especially important when first approaching healthcare professionals and seeking help as individuals will naturally have many fears and concerns. Kay Jamison (1995, p. 84) recounts aspects in her therapist's manner which helped to soothe her feelings of terror when making first contact:

I was – for the first time in my life – shaking with fear. I shook for what he might be able to tell me and I shook for what he might not be able to tell me … My psychiatrist sat me down and said something reassuring. I have completely forgotten what it was – and I am sure it was as much the manner in which it was said as the actual words – but slowly a tiny, very tiny, bit of light drifted into my dark and frightened mind.

This illustrates how effective and soothing the therapist's manner of conducting themselves can be and reflects the facilitative approach advocated by Rogers (1961). The feeling a person gets about their therapist will influence the degree to which they are able to engage. Talking about and sharing personal experiences, thoughts, feelings or impulses will be scary especially with the associated worries and concerns over how this will be responded to. This points to the essence of psychotherapeutic work and the importance of feeling safe, supported, contained, acknowledged and attended even when most distressed. A personal narrative illustrating the beneficial and healing potential states:

Psychotherapy heals. It makes sense of the confusion, reins in the terrifying thoughts and feelings, returns some control and opens the possibility of learning from it all.

Jamison (1995, p. 88)

This narrative illustrates key ways in which psychotherapy can help, especially in relation to the development of personal autonomy. Developing personal control creates hope and the belief that change can be affected. There are also reflections here upon the sense of order being brought to the 'chaos' and disorder with which one is struggling with.

Research by Jones et al. (2011) suggests that psycho-education, relapse prevention and recovery are all key aspects of psychological treatment for bipolar. Daggenvoorde and Goossens (2013) show that in the recovery process of individuals with bipolar, the development and use of a relapse prevention plan is an important tool in helping them to regain control. The element of control and personal responsibility taking is present in the four themes identified by Todd et al. (2012) with regard to psychotherapeutic approaches and recovery:

1. Recovery is not about being symptom-free.
2. Recovery requires taking responsibility for your own wellness.
3. Self-management: building on existing techniques.
4. Overcoming barriers to recovery: negativity, stigma and taboo.

This outlines the importance of involving the person actively within their own care and developing a sense of self-management and control.

Bernhard's (2010) study examined the use of cognitive-psycho-educative group therapy for individuals with bipolar after an acute episode. The initial results demonstrated satisfaction with a significant reduction of depressive symptoms, an improvement of global functioning and enhanced knowledge about bipolar. Berk et al. (2010) recommend the use of psycho-education to help clarify how medicines work. This will be helpful although healthcare professionals need to be mindful of what the tensions and potential problems are for each person. It means acknowledging what an individual receiving this form of treatment experiences within their internal frame of reference and why clear advice from professionals is not adhered to. The consequences of poorly managing one's symptoms can be very severe although for those concerned what they are experiencing within the here and now can overshadow this.

MEDICATION

In a study by Maczka et al. (2010), pharmacotherapy was regarded by service users and psychiatrists to be the most important intervention for bipolar treatment. The main pharmaceutical agents used in treating mood disorders are lithium, sodium valproate, olanzapine, carbamazepine and lamotrigine (Mind, 2013). Lithium has been used as a mood stabiliser for around 50 years. It requires regular blood tests and long-term use can affect the kidneys or the thyroid gland (RCP, 2012). Studies indicate beneficial results from the use of lithium for treating acute bipolar depression (Goodwin and Jamison, 1990) and acute mania (Levine and Chengappa, 2009). There have also been reported anti-suicidal effects from long-term lithium treatment (Baldessarii et al., 2003; Goodwin et al., 2003). Those prescribed medication will have their own individual feelings about taking it including fears around the loss of creativity. Blogger Shawn Maxam (2011) explains how being 'normal' with the aid of medication removed the 'advantages' of being bipolar. He recounts the detrimental impact upon his ability to be creative and write musical or poetic compositions which he felt particularly unsettled by as it is his art which he feels defined by as a person. This personal reflection illustrates a dilemma facing those with bipolar where 'normality' can come at a cost to one's creative and expressive ability. The difficulty here is in making comparisons to how a person feels when one's mood is elevated, and the senses are much more finely tuned. Whilst medication therapy offers a crucial lifeline for many people with bipolar regular maintenance and continued compliance can be problematic. Partial or non-adherence to medication in individuals with bipolar can have serious consequences including an exacerbation of symptoms and increased risk of suicide (Vieta et al., 2012). There are a number of factors affecting individuals' ability to take medication as prescribed including impaired judgement, rapidly fluctuating moods and the long-term nature of living with mood instability (Vega Perez et al., 2012). Lack of medication routines, unsupportive social networks, insufficient illness knowledge and treatment access problems may likewise affect overall adherence (Berk et al., 2010). The issues raised here are significant as a person's ability and desire to maintain routine medication regimes will fluctuate. It may also be affected by personal feelings about the effectiveness of this form of treatment. Vieta et al. (2012) found that many individuals who deteriorate after stopping medication do not attribute this to non-adherence. This fits in with some individuals' beliefs that medication is unnecessary and has no daily benefit (Devulapalli et al., 2010). In a number of these instances, non-compliance can be linked with alternative approaches being sought such as self-medication. External factors will also play a key part as Darling et al.'s (2008) study found that those adherent to medication had fewer health problems and more resources for coping with stress, possessed a stronger belief that their own behaviours controlled their health status and had higher life contentment compared to non-adherent participants.

A core factor influencing compliance concerns the problem of side effects (Sajatovic et al., 2011). An illustration of the associated physical side effects with lithium is given in Figure 5.5. The Bipolar UK's e-community has a range of discussion threads addressing daily problems faced by those prescribed medication and includes

- Starting new tablets and feeling very drowsy and irritable
- Concerned about other's reaction when picking up medication from the chemists
- Worries about taking medication whilst trying for a baby and being pregnant.
- Not wanting 'high'/happy feelings to go away

These discussion topics illustrate clearly some of the day-to-day issues and worries around taking medication. There are concerns here about side effects as well as the

---

- Feeling thirsty
- Passing more urine than usual
- Gaining weight
- Having blurred vision
- Feeling slight muscle weakness
- Experiencing occasional diarrhoea
- Acquiring fine trembling of the hands
- Feeling of being mildly ill

How would you feel about this information if you were prescribed Lithium?

Figure 5.5 Lithium – side effects. (From British National Formulary, BNF, 2015, https://www.medicinescomplete.com/mc/bnf/current/, accessed 17 June, 2015.)

affirmation given of having mental health difficulties and the potential stigmatising responses from others. The last discussion topic listed (*not wanting 'high'/happy feelings to go away*) demonstrates the strong desire individuals can have of prolonging one's mood state and avoiding becoming depressed. This worry is reflected through multiple narratives where people strive to hold on to a state in which they relate feeling productive, 'alive' and vibrant. The degree to which individuals are affected by this will vary from person to person with some more accepting of the effects of medication. The actor Richard Dreyfus uses the analogy of a letterbox to explain the effects that taking lithium has had on him, with the top and bottom of his perceptual world being removed leaving a narrow space within which he can live in (Wilson, 2006). Whilst feeling restrictive, he stated that for him taking medication helped him reclaim both his life and career. Individuals evidently have very varied experiences and feelings about taking medication and cover a whole spectrum. Understanding and awareness as to what this experience entails or means is essential for those prescribing or maintaining people on medication regimes.

IN-PATIENT CARE

For a number of people with bipolar, there will be occasions when hospitalisation becomes necessary. The experience of hospital care will depend upon a variety of factors such as whether it is their first time, the level and type of support available, their current mental health state and the environmental climate of the unit admitted to. This occurs at a time when individuals already feel out of control, enduring lives which are feeling increasingly chaotic or distressing. This will be a time of feeling vulnerable, frightened and helpless, desperately needing support. It was with feelings similar to this that Michelle (DBSA, 2015) entered hospital:

> Once there, I had the same problem I'd been having with everyone else. I couldn't communicate, I was suspicious of everyone's motives, and I was very scared. I screamed at them that I didn't want to be committed. One nurse tried to explain that I was being admitted, not committed, but I was convinced that I'd be locked up and never come out.

The fears can evidently create fantasies about the meaning of one's admission. These need addressing in order for hospital to offer one of its most beneficial functions – a much needed refuge, a place of safety where equilibrium can be restored. This is reflected by Hornbacher (2008) regarding months in her life to which she has little or no recollection. Her time in hospital gradually enabled her to 'find herself' and emerge from her fugue-type state. The support provided can literally be a lifesaver when chaotic thoughts and behaviour spiral out of control. For Liz Miller (Wilson, 2006) being sectioned and hospitalised represented a turning point for her, providing her with space to make sense of what she was experiencing and opportunities to begin taking control over her life.

For a number of individuals with bipolar the process can feel cyclical with a series of 'breakdowns' and readmissions experienced. Neil Walton writes about his fourth period of hospitalisation following his deteriorating mental health state and being embroiled in a series of public incidents:

> There were some colourful exchanges of language and then I was helped to
> the floor by an unknown assailant ... From my resting point I saw the familiar
> sight of a flashing blue light ... Our destination, although I didn't know it at the
> time, was a psychiatric unit called Naseberry Court.

Walton (2007, p. 179)

Although writing with humour and warmth his account depicts his sense of resignation at requiring further periods of in-patient care. He does however go on to stress the essential support provided which enabled him to reacquire his sense of equilibrium and feeling of stability. Having the knowledge that one has a place of safety to retreat to when needed is shown through a number of narratives to be extremely reassuring, something which is vitally important when feeling hopeless or out of control. A major concern however relates to the level of distress and chaotic experience that is endured by some people before effective support is obtained. The narratives reflected in Section 1: Experiencing bipolar, for instance, highlight the severe impact upon a person's thoughts and behaviour from both depressed and elevated mood states.

Whilst hospitalisation can be necessary and life-saving this experience can for some be perceived as humiliating, depersonalising and shameful. A Time to Change (2014e) blogger reflects:

> The me that once sat quivering in the corner of the locked solitary confinement
> room, or that once hid in unwashed pyjamas and a dirty dressing gown – the
> belt taken away by the nurses because I pose a risk to myself and other patients.

This extract is illustrative in terms of reminding us that such experiences can leave an indelible mark on people. Likewise, Ruth (Mind, 2014b) recalls:

> I eventually became so manic that I had to be pinned down by four people who
> stuck a needle in my bottom. The next few days were a complete haze. One
> thing I can remember is not being able to lift my head off the hospital bed and
> drooling like a boxer dog.

The recollection of how one felt when in need of help as well as the way in which care was delivered can be difficult to feel alright with. Factors strongly expressed through these narrative concern feelings of powerlessness and the loss of dignity. It is therefore imperative that health carers are mindful of what this experience might feel like for those concerned and take care to properly support people through such experiences.

Whilst being in hospital can feel reassuring and safe returning home can cause extreme worry feeling as if one is emerging from a cocoon. For Johnston (2002), leaving the protective shield that the ward had provided her with left her feeling exposed and vulnerable. Similarly, Adam Ant (Goddard, 2006) states:

> I returned home after three months. I had no life in me and felt totally deflated. I
> finally went back to work, but my confidence had been knocked sideways. I put
> on four stone due to my medication and battled every day to build my strength.
> I felt a different person and became very depressed.

This shows how hard it can be to 'restart' oneself as after all, many people will be returning to lives which had become entangled with conflict or distress and where one's behaviour had impacted upon others. Recommencing activities and occupation as well as re-establishing relationships can provoke much unease and discomfort. It highlights a clear need to prepare people for this transition and to support them with regaining their confidence and ability to cope.

CREATIVE APPROACHES

There are a variety of creative activities and artistic interventions which have proven helpful with the experience of bipolar including art, music and sport. Henley (2007) reports upon a successfully trialled art therapy intervention with children and adolescents with bipolar. Art can be diverting and relaxing as well as providing a potent means of self-expression. This can be seen with Wheatley's (2012) narrative around his use of art, including doodles as a means of externalising his feelings and enabling insights into his condition.

Bednarz and Nikkel (1992) detail the value of music in helping improve the quality of life of young adults with bipolar and substance abuse. The beneficial qualities are also related by other narratives including that of blogger Karl Shallowhorn (BP Hope, 2015, bphope.com for bipolar Blogger & Director, Mental Health Association, Buffalo, NY) who shares the important function music provides when he is feeling depressed listing a number of artists and whose music 'speaks to his soul'.

Another important intervention helping with bipolar symptoms is exercise. This is especially related to low mood through offering a diversion from negative thoughts (Mynors-Wallis et al., 2000) and changes in endorphin and monoamine concentrations (Leith, 1994). It also helps counter weight gain which can be linked to a number of drugs used in the treatment of bipolar (National Collaborating Centre for Mental Health, 2006). Nanda et al.'s (2012) study examined the current literature on the effect of yoga on bipolar perinatal populations finding reductions in anxiety and depressive symptoms, cortisol levels and an increase in quality of life after yoga therapy. Mills (Lindsay and Mills, 2013) raises a point of note relating to different responses depending upon whether his mood state was depressed or elevated. He found exercise beneficial in reducing stress and boosting low mood however:

> If I am hypomanic, I find that exercise does not alleviate the stress as effectively. My thoughts would be racing and I would walk or swim faster and faster and find that I was no more relaxed nor better able to cope with stress than before I exercised. In fact I was more reactive.

Support can also be obtained from some fairly unique and surprising sources. Becky (Mind, 2014c) blogs about creatively reframing her bipolar experience. One approach involves relating her symptoms and experiences to characters she has watched in television comedy sitcoms. She has also found constructing an imaginary dating profile for her medication side effects helpful. This is obviously a very personal approach which works for her. Attention is evidently needed to work with each individual to find what works for them no matter how unusual or abstract. It can even include small interventions, elements which collectively can provide optimism, symptom relief or hope. A Time to Change (2014b) blogger relates the small things that been instrumental in her recovery which include buying her favourite cake for lunchtimes, getting lifts home from work on dark and wet days or being texted by friends inquiring after her on days she was upset:

> I never found this intrusive and they helped me open up and realise that I could be a teacher and be bipolar and that it really is the small things that can pull someone out of a dark place.

It is evident from the information covered here that creative activities can significantly enhance a person's well-being. There are however issues to consider concerning variable responses to the same interventions, depending upon whether a person's mood is elevated or depressed.

PEER SUPPORT

> How important do you feel support is from peers (others experiencing bipolar)?

A crucial need for those with bipolar or any other mental health difficulty is a sense of engagement with people who understand (Rethink Mental Illness, 2015). This can be found with those who are experiencing similar issues and who it is felt will better comprehend what is encountered. The engagement with peers illustrates a reciprocal benefit involving the help which can be received as well as the support which can be offered to others. Self-help groups feature strongly here with both face-to-face and online contact indicated. A number of postings in Bipolar UK's (2013) e-community reflected how crucially important it felt to have others to connect with and share one's experience with. This illustrates the need for such forms of support given the level of distress felt. As seen throughout this chapter, there are times when people feel exceedingly fragile, raw and vulnerable. Fears around potentially discriminatory or hostile reactions make it hard to open up and share thoughts and feelings. This is compounded by a sense of feeling 'different' which creates added difficulty. The peer community provides a resource of likeminded people, individuals who can be trusted and who it is felt will react sensitively and with understanding. This is clearly borne out by the supportive nature of the Bipolar UK's discussion forum postings. It is also noticeable within other online forums that the same people asking for support and help are at other times offering support to others. This illustrates the dual roles that a person can operate in relating to others from positions of vulnerability and resilience. The value of what is offered is highlighted in responses as being instrumental in a person's ongoing recovery and sense of coping.

A very important peer resource is Time to Change's 'voice of experience'. This initiative engages people with mental health problems in answering questions about their mental health experience. One member (Time to Change, 2014f) states:

> For nearly ten years I'd been going round with this hidden secret and I found by attending these events and especially talking with the other people with experience of mental health problems, that that burden has gone. It has been very

liberating and I think that whereas before I might have avoided talking about it at all costs, I now wouldn't mind so much.

This narrative is heartening to read and the sense of liberation gained through talking with others illustrates the benefits in feeling accepted and dispelling some of the associated myths. An increasingly popular format for sharing experience and connecting with peers is through writing blogs. Katie (Mind, 2014a) states:

I find writing and blogging to be therapeutic and it's an easier way to explain how I feel.

It also appears very beneficial to others given the nature of the replies to her narratives.

The contact with peers can be widened to incorporate other examples such as engagement through in-patient care. Michelle (DBSA, 2015) highlights the vital support received from peers whilst in hospital:

I got the best support from other patients on the unit. I had something in common with most of them, and with long stretches of time between groups and educational sessions, we learned a lot about each other. My roommate was especially kind, considering it took me several more nights to actually sleep.

This was clearly important especially at a time when feeling especially vulnerable and anxious. It reflects the other narratives addressed earlier in highlighting how valuable connecting with peers can be. There are some very positive benefits received through having space to express oneself freely, feel accepted and being able to receive and offer help.

FAMILY AND FRIENDS

A significant source of support concerns one's family and friends. This is confirmed by a blogger who regards them as her most important resource with her mother in particular seen as being her 'rock' (Time to Change, 2014g). Similarly, another blogger expresses the support she received from her family:

A large chunk of my life has been a total mess. When I was ill my moods were all over the place and my life seemed like a pit of hell that would never end. I was in pain and simply existing became such a challenge; a challenge that I wanted to give up on. What made this pain bearable were the people I had around me. I was fighting a battle, but I wasn't fighting it alone. I was surrounded by love and support every step of the way. My family were by my side throughout.

Time to Change (2014h)

These narratives highlight the value in having a 'constant' with which to anchor oneself to. Having a *rock* or family member by one's side provides a reassuring presence, a comforting source of support to counter the disrupted and tempestuous experience with which one is struggling. As seen within discussion threads in discussion forums, family members can provide a vital function of notifying a person if, for example, their behaviour is changing and becoming more erratic. It is clear that having people to whom one can go to is important. What comes across powerfully from these narratives relates to the importance of knowing that others care, that there are people out there looking out for one and to whom one can turn to if in need.

SECTION 3: LIVING WELL

Interview narratives

I have a lot of awareness about the triggers that are good for me or not so good for me.

I worked for Mind for 10 years and got a lot out of it besides giving other people help … it gives you the confidence in your own ability to stay well.

If we feel that I am going a little bit high, I'll hand over my credit card and cheque book just in case.

I find that the more knowledge and information you have, the more chance you have of working through things and supporting yourself.

I suppose it's [bipolar] part of me, and although at times it's distressing for me and my family in some ways, the experiences I've had will have changed me in a positive way … I have become a better person through the experiences I've had.

The sections earlier have been concerned with the experience of living with bipolar and the interventions used to treat it. A wide range of issues have been addressed primarily relating troubling symptoms, which lie at one end of the struggling – coping continuum. At the other end we can embrace concepts such as living well and recovery, a point at which individuals are able to cope and take charge of their lives. The multifaceted elements of this condition are eloquently expressed by Jamison (1995, p. 218):

> So why would I want anything to do with this illness? I believe as a result of it I have felt more things, more deeply … Depressed, I have crawled on my hands and knees in order to get across a room and have done it month after month. But, normal or manic, I have run faster, thought faster, and loved faster than most I know … Even when I have been most psychotic – delusional, hallucinating, frenzied – I have been aware of finding new corners of my mind and heart. Some of those corners were incredible and beautiful and took my breath away and made me feel as though I could die right then and the images would sustain me.

This illustrates moments of well-being whilst in the midst of symptoms. There is a sense here of really feeling 'in the world' with a more exquisite appreciation of experiences and perceived stimuli. Other narratives highlight well-being in connection with *recovery* and the beneficial position people find themselves in. As Helen (Mind, 2014d) states:

My life is full and fulfilling. I have a job, a husband and friends. I have interests and passions in which I am fully engaged. I have built a sense of well-being that centres around doing things I believe in and value, connecting with people who inspire me and who I care about. I give what I can to those around me and the world I live in. I try new things, developing new knowledge, skills and perspectives and a better awareness and appreciation of the world in which I live.

This is a person living with bipolar or more accurately living well with bipolar. It demonstrates that fulfilling, productive and happy lives are possible even though there may be times when things become fragmented and chaotic. It importantly shows the position of resilience which can be attained as well as learning attained through working through one's difficulties. This can be seen with the following narrative:

A *mental illness* with the effects that *Bipolar Disorder* has will force perspective on a person … The illness has taught me to not judge, to consider the root cause of people's actions … I have learnt, the hard way, that to be forgiving of others' indiscretions, their aggressions, is a hugely worthwhile discipline. I am a fighter. After each break down, or set-back, I recrystallise, and attempt to rebuild *relationships* with family, lovers and friends, forge ahead with my work. I'll never give up and for this I am proud of myself.

Time to Change (2012b)

The statement here shows a very real position of strength and determination challenging many stereotypical notions of people with mental health difficulties.

A Time to Change (2014a) blogger reflects upon the lost years in her life, a time spent struggling to cope with self-destructive rage. She has subsequently reached a position of acceptance, acknowledging herself as a person of two extremes. This has enabled her to feel more optimistic and able to face her future with

Positivity, creativity and love. I will fight the inevitable relapses that are sure to hit as life steers its precarious course.

This narrative reflects a sense of realism accepting the fact that life will not necessarily be free from difficulty. It also shows a degree of resilience, understanding and hope.

The issue concerning what it means to be bipolar is a difficult concept to encapsulate. It clearly means something very different to each person. A fascinating question raised during Stephen Fry's *The Secret Life of the Manic Depressive* documentary (Wilson, 2006) concerned whether or not those affected would 'push the button' and exchange their condition for 'normality'. There were some respondents who clearly would 'push the button' on account of the devastation to their lives which were experienced as tormented and blighted existence. Surprisingly, this was not a universal response with some people highlighting how their bipolar had helped to define who they were or how they had developed on account of their experience and how consequently they would not push the button. A point which need stating here is that answers to this question will no doubt vary according to one's fluctuating mood state although, nevertheless, illustrate how individuals in recovery can reach a point of acceptance with what they have experienced. For Michelle (DBSA, 2015) acceptance meant acknowledging the need to take personal responsibility and learning ways of self-monitoring and regulating her care. She was also able to reframe her experience in an adaptive and hopeful light:

> I used to be really ashamed that I'd had to be hospitalized, but eleven years later, it's a lot easier to see the benefits of the whole experience. I couldn't have gotten well on my own. With the severity of my symptoms, it had been wise to get me out of the chaotic world I lived in and into a place where the only thing I had to worry about was stabilizing my mood, which at the time was a full-time job.

The narratives shown within this section therefore provide effective role models with whom others can be inspired by. These are people who have endured severe distress and difficulty in their lives yet been able to reach a point of resolution and coping.

A final point concerns that of staying well and avoiding relapse. A study by Simhandl et al. (2014) found 204 out of 300 patients (with bipolar I and bipolar II) relapsing within 4 years after discharge from hospital. They provide advice which includes the following:

- Keep up with your treatment (i.e. medication and psychotherapy).
- Take bipolar seriously.
- Change your lifestyle to create a more stable environment.
- Reduce your stress.
- Learn about the prodromal (early) symptoms of a bipolar episode.
- Track your mood and watch for subtle changes.
- Learn bipolar coping skills.
- Don't take you wellness for granted – work at keeping it every day.

The ability to act upon this advice and to maintain changes will obviously vary from person to person and be influenced by one's available network of support. It does though provide opportunities for self-management and living well with bipolar.

REFERENCES

Adams, B. (2003). *The Pits and the Pendulum: A Life with Bipolar Disorder.* Jessica Kingsley Publishers: London, UK.

Bailey, S. and Shooter, M. (2009). *The Young Mind: An Essential Guide to Mental Health for Young Adults, Parents and Teachers.* Bantam Press: London, UK.

Baldessarii, R., Tondo, L. and Hennen, J. (2003). Lithium treatment and suicide risk in major affective disorders: Update and new findings. *The Journal of Clinical Psychiatry.* 64(5), 44–52.

BBC (2010). EastEnders' bipolar story helps young seek advice. http://www.bbc.co.uk, accessed 18 April, 2014.

Bednarz, L.F. and Nikkel, B. (1992). The role of music therapy in the treatment of young adults diagnosed with mental illness and substance abuse. *Music Therapy Perspectives.* 10(1), 21–26.

Berk, L., Hallam, K.T., Colom, F., Vieta, E., Hasty, M., Macneil, C. and Berk, M. (2010). Enhancing medication adherence in patients with bipolar disorder. *Human Psychopharmacology*. 25(1), 1–16.

Bernhard, B. (2010). Cognitive-psychoeducative group therapy for patients with bipolar disorder. *European Psychiatry*. 25(1), 21.

Bipolar UK (2013). E-Community. http://www.bipolaruk.org.uk, accessed 12 July, 2015.

Bipolar UK (2015). Information. http://www.bipolaruk.org.uk, accessed 12 July, 2015.

Bowden, C.L. (2009). Diagnosis and impact of bipolar depression. *The Journal of Clinical Psychiatry*. 70(9), e32.

BP Hope (2014). Don't break the bank: Bipolar & overspending. http://www.bphope.com, accessed 8 October, 2015.

BP Hope (2015). Bipolar, RUSH, and the healing power of music. http://www.bphope.com, accessed 8 October, 2015.

British National Formulary (2015). BNF. https://www.medicinescomplete.com/mc/bnf/current/, accessed 17 June, 2015.

Cheney, T. (2008). *Manic*. Harper Element: London, UK.

Daggenvoorde, T.H. and Goossens, P.J.J. (2013). Regained control: A phenomenological study of the use of a relapse prevention plan by patients with a bipolar disorder. *Perspectives in Psychiatric Care*. 49(4), 235–242.

Darling, C.A., Olmstead, S.B., Lund, V.E. and Fairclough, J.F. (2008). Bipolar disorder: Medication adherence and life contentment. *Archives of Psychiatric Nursing*. 22(3), 113–126.

DBSA (2015). Michelle's Story. http://www.dbsalliance.org, accessed 22 August, 2015.

Devulapalli, K.K., Ignacio, R.V., Weiden, P., Cassidy, K.A., Williams, T.D., Safavi, R. et al. (2010). Why do persons with bipolar disorder stop their medication? *Psychopharmacology Bulletin*. 43(3), 5–14.

Eden, G. (2007). Manic depression. In N. Carver, J. Morrison, N. Clibbens and T. Simpson (Eds.), *Greater Goings On … (Than You Would Ever Guess …)* (p. 35). Asylum Publishing: Sheffield, England.

Finseth, P.I., Morken, G., Andreassen, O.A., Malt, U.F. and Vaaler, A.E. (2012). Risk factors related to lifetime suicide attempts in acutely admitted bipolar disorder inpatients. *Bipolar Disorders*. 14(7), 727–734.

Goddard, S. (2006). *Stand and Deliver*. Sidgwick & Jackson: London, UK.

Goodwin, F., Fireman, B., Simo, G., Hukoler, E., Lee, J. and Revicki, D. (2003). Suicide risk in bipolar disorder during treatment with lithium and divalproex. *Journal of the American Medical Association*. 290(11), 1467–1473.

Goodwin, F.K. and Jamison, K.R. (1990). *Manic-Depressive Illness: Bipolar Disorders and Recurrent Depression*. Oxford University Press: Oxford, UK.

Henley, D. (2007). Naming the enemy: An art therapy intervention for children with bipolar and comorbid disorders. *Art Therapy*. 24(3), 104–110.

Hornbacher, M. (2008). *Madness – A Bipolar Life*. Houghton Mifflin: New York.

Jamison, K. (1995). *An Unquiet Mind: A Memoir of Moods and Madness*. Vintage Books: New York.

Johnston, S. (2002). *The Naked Bird Watcher* (2nd ed.). The Cairn: Helensburgh, Scotland.

Jones, S., Deville, M., Mayes, D. and Lobban, F. (2011). Self-management in bipolar disorder: The story so far. *Journal of Mental Health*. 20(6), 583–592.

Jones, S., Hayward, P. and Lam, D. (2009). *Coping with Bipolar Disorder. A CBT Informed Guide to Living with Manic Depression*. One World: Oxford, UK.

Ketter, T.A. (2010). Diagnostic features, prevalence, and impact of bipolar disorder. *The Journal of Clinical Psychiatry*. 71(6), e14.

Lakhani, N. (2008). Spending sprees plunge mental health patients into chronic debt. http://www.independent.co.uk, accessed 23 September, 2014.

Leith, L.M. (1994). *Foundations of Exercise and Mental Health*. Fitness Information Technology: Morgantown, WV.

Levine, J. and Chengappa, R. (2009). Lithium in the treatment of bipolar disorder. In L. Yatham and V. Kusumakar (Eds.), *Bipolar Disorder – A Clinician's Guide to Treatment* (2nd ed., pp. 259–294). Routledge: London, UK.

Lindsay, A.C. and Mills, M.J. (2013). Physical activity, bipolar disorder and me. *International Journal of Psychosocial Rehabilitation*. 18(1), 125–132.

Lowry, M. (1947). *Under the Volcano*. Penguin: London, UK.

Maczka, G., Siwek, M., Skalski, M., Grabski, B. and Dudek, D. (2010). Patients' and doctors' attitudes towards bipolar disorder – Do we share our beliefs? *Archives of Psychiatry and Psychotherapy*. 12(2), 43–50.

Maxam, S. (2011). David Foster Wallace – Creativity killed the cat. http://goodmenproject.com, accessed 17 December, 2013.

Mind (2013). Bipolar. http://www.mind.org.uk, accessed 16 May, 2014.

Mind (2014a). Hearing voices with bipolar disorder. http://www.mind.org.uk, accessed 12 January, 2015.

Mind (2014b). My battle with bipolar and medication. http://www.mind.org.uk, accessed 12 January, 2015.

Mind (2014c). How sitcoms help my bipolar disorder. http://www.mind.org.uk, accessed 12 January, 2015.

Mind (2014d). What does depression feel like? http://www.mind.org.uk, accessed 12 January, 2015.

Morris, G. (2006). *Mental Health Issues and the Media*. Routledge: London, UK.

Morris, R. (2008). *Don't Wait for Me*. Mainstream Publishing: Edinburgh, Scotland.

Mynors-Wallis, L.M., Gath, D.H. and Baker, F. (2000). Randomised controlled trial and cost analysis of problems solving treatment for emotional disorders given by community nurses in primary care. *British Medical Journal*. 320, 26–30.

Nanda, A., Abizadeh, J. and Misri, S. (March 2012). Yoga as a complementary therapy for the improvement of quality of life in perinatal women with bipolar disorder. Paper presented at *Fifth Biennial Conference of the International Society for Bipolar Disorders*, Istanbul, Turkey.

National Collaborating Centre for Mental Health (2006). The management of bipolar disorder in adults, children and adolescents, in primary and secondary care. NICE Clinical Guidelines, No. 38. http://www.ncbi.nlm.nih.gov, accessed 7 February, 2014.

RCP (2012). Bipolar. http://www.rcpsych.ac.uk, accessed 12 July, 2015.

Rethink Mental Illness (2015). Staying well with bipolar. http://www.rethink.org, accessed 28 September, 2015.

Rogers, C. (1961). *On Becoming a Person*. Constable & Robinson: London, UK.

Sajatovic, M., Levin, J., Fuentes-Casiano, E., Cassidy, K.A., Tatsuoka, C. and Jenkins, J.H. (2011). Illness experience and reasons for nonadherence among individuals with bipolar disorder who are poorly adherent with medication. *Comprehensive Psychiatry*. 52(3), 280–287.

Simhandl, C., König, B. and Amann, B.L. (2014). A prospective 4-year naturalistic follow-up of treatment and outcome of 300 bipolar I and II patients. *The Journal of Clinical Psychiatry*. 75(3), 254–262.

Song, J.Y., Yu, H.Y., Kim, S.H., Hwang, S.S.H., Cho, H.S., Kim, Y.S. et al. (2012). Assessment of risk factors related to suicide attempts in patients with bipolar disorder. *Journal of Nervous and Mental Disease*. 200(11), 978–984.

Swann, A.C. (2010). The Strong relationship between bipolar and substance-use disorder: Mechanisms and treatment implications. *Annals of the New York Academy of Sciences*. 1187, 276–293.

Thangavelu, K., Morriss, R. and Howard, R. (2012). Suicidality in bipolar affective disorder the nature of impulsivity and impulse control disorders – A cross sectional controlled study. *European Psychiatry*. 27, 1.

Time to Change (2012a). Personal narrative. http://www.time-to-change.org.uk, accessed 20 August, 2015.

Time to Change (2012b). Personal narrative. http://www.time-to-change.org.uk, accessed 20 August, 2015.

Time to Change (2014a). Personal narrative. http://www.time-to-change.org.uk, accessed 20 August, 2015.

Time to Change (2014b). Personal narrative. http://www.time-to-change.org.uk, accessed 20 August, 2015.

Time to Change (2014c). Personal narrative. http://www.time-to-change.org.uk, accessed 20 August, 2015.

Time to Change (2014d). Personal narrative. http://www.time-to-change.org.uk, accessed 20 August, 2015.

Time to Change (2014e). Personal narrative. http://www.time-to-change.org.uk, accessed 20 August, 2015.

Time to Change (2014f). Personal narrative. http://www.time-to-change.org.uk, accessed 20 August, 2015.

Time to Change (2014g). Personal narrative. http://www.time-to-change.org.uk, accessed 20 August, 2015.

Time to Change (2014h). Personal narrative. http://www.time-to-change.org.uk, accessed 20 August, 2015.

Todd, N.J., Jones, S.H. and Lobban, F.A. (2012). "Recovery" in bipolar disorder: How can service users be supported through a self-management intervention? A qualitative focus group study. *Journal of Mental Health*. 21(2), 114–126.

Tracy, N. (2014). Bipolar burble. http://natashatracy.com, accessed 16 June, 2016.

Vega Perez, P., Ruiz de Azua Garcia, S., Barbeito Resa, S., Gonzalez-Ortega, I., Ugart, A., Karim Haidar, M. et al. (2012). Why do male bipolar patients not comply with treatment? *European Neuropsychopharmacology*. 22, 282–283.

Vieta, E., Azorin, J.M., Bauer, M., Frangou, S., Perugi, G., Martinez, G. and Schreiner, A. (2012). Psychiatrists' perceptions of potential reasons for non- and partial adherence to medication: Results of a survey in bipolar disorder from eight European countries. *Journal of Affective Disorders*. 143, 125–130.

Walton, N. (2007). *Bipolar Expedition*. Chipmunkapublishing: Essex, England.

Ward, T.D. (2011). The lived experience of adults with bipolar disorder and comorbid substance use disorder. *Issues in Mental Health Nursing*. 32(1), 20–27.

Wheatley, D.N. (2012). *BipolART: Art and Bipolar Disorder: A Personal Perspective*. Springer Science: New York.

Wilson, R. (2006). *The Secret Life of the Manic Depressive*. IWC Media: Glasgow, Scotland.

Woolf, V. (1953). *A Writer's Diary; Virginia Woolf*. Hogarth Press: London, UK.

Yeloglu, C.H., Guveli, H., Sarp, K., Bahceci, B. and Hocaoglu, C. (April 2011). Treatment of bipolar disorder in adolescents: A case report. Paper presented at *Fourth International Congress on Psychopharmacology*, Antalya, Turkey.

Your Stories (2014). Maxine Wade. http://www.leedsandyorkpft.nhs.uk.

Your Voices (2012). Tricia Thorp. http://www.leedsandyorkpft.nhs.uk.

6

'There's a storm inside'
Living with altered reality

INTRODUCTION

This chapter is about the experience of altered reality linked with mental health states such as psychosis and schizophrenia. When considering what the concept of *altered reality* means, it is important to first define *reality*, which according to the *Oxford English Dictionary* (2015) is

> the quality of being real or having an actual existence or correspondence to fact; truth.

This raises a number of issues as existence can be created internally or through shared consensus with others. Shared consensus though can differ widely concerning different political, religious or personal affiliations. There is also a historical dimension concerning what is deemed to be *real* with new knowledge replacing previously held facts, for example, the old belief amongst sailors that the world was flat. A key aspect concerns acceptance and validation of experience by sizeable or influential groups. An illustration of this concerns the apparitions of the Virgin Mary experienced by a 14-year-old girl, Bernadette Soubirous. This experience was taken seriously by the Catholic church resulting in the establishment of a major shrine at Lourdes. Societal views about people who see the world differently to the majority are often far from supportive though. The ex-sports presenter David Icke, for example, has been met with scorn, derision and abuse within the media for his controversial and 'unworldly' beliefs about *reptilian beings* yet at the same time sells out major world venues with his shows and hosts a discussion forum containing millions of posts. It is important to acknowledge the broad variation in responses to different people's views and experiences. Creative and artistic individuals can be praised for their abstract or creative view of the world, and indeed may even purposely seek altered states through chemical means. Notable examples include the writers Carlos Castenada and Aldous Huxley or the Pink Floyd musician Syd Barrett. For some people, if supported by religious or political views their experiences can be regarded as visionary or even miraculous. The majority of people however who experience altered reality are dismissed, made fun of or abused and offered various interventions in an attempt to remove or change their worldly views or experiences. This chapter is mainly about this latter group, individuals who have their altered states of reality classified through medical diagnoses such as psychosis and schizophrenia. It is important to note

131

though that psychotic symptoms can occur in a number of other mental health states, for example, depression and dementia.

WHAT IS PSYCHOSIS/SCHIZOPHRENIA?

What do you understand by the terms 'psychosis' and 'schizophrenia'?

Psychosis describes hearing or seeing things, or holding unusual beliefs that other people do not share or involve a 'break from reality'. Common examples include hearing voices or believing that people are trying to do one harm (Rethink Mental Illness, 2014). Psychotic symptoms can be linked to a variety of psychiatric and physical health states (see Figure 6.1).

One of the main conditions linked here is schizophrenia which can be regarded as chronic, severe, and disabling. People with this condition may experience hallucinations or believe that others are able to read their minds, control their thoughts or have intent to harm them. The causes can be linked to genetic, environmental, psychological or biological factors (NIMH, 2015). Around one in every hundred people is affected with schizophrenia which usually starts in early adulthood (Rethink Mental Illness, 2014).

SCHIZOPHRENIA/PSYCHOSIS: POSITIVE AND NEGATIVE SYMPTOMS

The symptoms of schizophrenia can be divided into 'positive' symptoms (additional to those things experienced by the general population) and 'negative' symptoms (preventing individuals from doing what other people do).

Psychosis relates to a set of symptoms that can be linked with:

- Schizophrenia
- Bipolar disorder
- Schizoaffective disorder
- Drug-induced psychosis
- Psychotic depression
- Postnatal (puerperal) psychosis
- Personality disorder
- Organic psychosis
- Delusional disorder
- Reaction psychosis/brief psychotic episode – can follow major stressful event or trauma

---

Figure 6.1 Conditions linked with psychosis. (From Rethink Mental Illness, Schizophrenia, 2014, https://www.rethink.org, accessed 18 November, 2014.)

POSITIVE SYMPTOMS

The terms 'positive symptoms' and 'psychosis' are generally used to describe the same symptoms and include

- Hallucinations
- Delusions
- Disorganised thinking

NEGATIVE SYMPTOMS

These symptoms involve loss of ability and enjoyment in life. They are much less dramatic than psychotic symptoms although can be perceived as more troubling and tend to be more persistent. They include (Rethink Mental Illness, 2014)

- Lack of motivation
- Slow movement
- Change in sleep patterns
- Poor grooming or hygiene
- Difficulty in planning and setting goals
- Not saying much
- Changes in body language
- Lack of eye contact
- Reduced range of emotions
- A tendency not to interact with other people
- Little interest in having hobbies
- Little interest in sex

WHAT IT IS NOT (MISCONCEPTIONS)

There are a number of commonly held misconceptions about mental health states particularly relating to psychosis and schizophrenia. One erroneous association relates to the belief that people with schizophrenia have a split personality which is simply not true (NHS Choices, 2014a). Another commonly held view concerns the heightened potential of violence even though the risk from people with psychosis and schizophrenia is significantly small (NIMH, 2015). The reality is that people with mental health problems including those experiencing psychosis are more at risk of harm and abuse from others than they are of posing a threat themselves (Morrall, 2000). These erroneous beliefs are largely fuelled by stereotypical and sensationalist types of media reporting and whilst increasing a product's commercial appeal, stigmatising and misleading messages are very damaging to people living with mental health problems (Morris, 2006). The popular film *Me, Myself and Irene* (Farrelly and Farrelly, 2000) portrayed both of the aforementioned misconceptions and was severely criticised by mental health charities including Mind. The main character's supposed diagnosis of *Advanced Delusionary Schizophrenia with Involuntary Narcissistic Rage* is totally misleading. A point missed by the many supporters of this film who describe it as hilarious and 'just harmless fun' is the negative impact caused by stigmatising messages such as this upon people living with mental health issues.

SECTION 1: EXPERIENCING PSYCHOSIS

FIRST EXPERIENCES

Interview narratives

When I actually became unwell or it was noticed that I was not my usual self I actually wasn't aware of it.

I'd go into the kitchen and start making a cup of tea and wander out and walk back in and start making a different cup of tea and eventually there was about 5 cups of tea in there.

I were in the back bedroom and it was just full of demons, black robed things all screaming kill yourself, you're going to be a dosser. You're never going to work again.

I think it's good to be able to have something [diagnosis] to help explain what's going on because it's a very confusing experience. The recognition that it's something that other people have experienced and that there's a set of common symptoms that you can identify with can be helpful.

I get shocked sometimes at other people's reactions.

[My voices] are people I know. I still get them from time to time but they are benign.

I was good at masking it [voice hearing] and hiding it. I was talking to them internally and I knew enough that they might think I was mad if I showed what I was doing.

The psychiatrist told me I was hearing voices which was strange because it doesn't do justice to the experience. The phrase 'hearing voices' does not go anywhere near it. It is like saying black and white is a rainbow.

I was talking really fast. I remember being quite hyperactive and hypersensitive to things that were going on. I wasn't sleeping and apart from being manic.

People point when I talk to myself and swear back at [the voices].

Things would take on a lot of significance so you could see something fairly normal like a bird flying or a message on somebody's T-shirt and it would directly be speaking to you.

The first realisation that a person might be experiencing mental health problems can be a confusing and traumatic time. The emergence of symptoms can be sudden or insidious, slowly developing towards a point whereby they cannot be ignored. Psychotic symptoms significantly affect people with all areas and spheres in their life impacted upon (Cook and Chambers, 2009; Lloyd et al., 2008). The first episode typically occurs between the ages of 15 and 30 years, a critical transitional period and a time of huge significance (Ballageer et al., 2005). The initial awareness that individuals have of altered thinking is no doubt a period of considerable distress. At first they may have little or no understanding about what is happening besides a growing awareness that 'something is wrong'. What exactly *is* seen as wrong will differ from person to person. Whilst there might be an awareness that one's internal thoughts and feelings seem to be at odds with those of others, the problems can be put down to alterations in self or seemingly erratic, persecutory and critical behaviour of others. It may be that the irrationality of one's thoughts, whilst being evidently noticeable to others, remains undetected by those affected. This brings a person into multiple points of conflict as they are unable to grasp why others cannot appreciate or comprehend what is *clearly* occurring to them. Alternatively, strange or irrational thoughts will be personally concerning and can lead to experiences being concealed from others or rationalised as a means of coping. Elyn Saks (2007, p. 48) vividly recounts the emerging fantasies and unreal thoughts she was experiencing to which other people were oblivious:

> No one looking at me would have known there was a storm going on inside. But there was a storm and it was horrible.

Trying to maintain the appearance of normality in order to protect oneself from others' judgements can be extremely stressful. This initial stage can be a bewildering, terrifying and isolatory experience as individuals struggle to make sense of what is happening internally for them. Whilst narratives predominantly document distressing experiences, for a small number of people symptoms are not negatively regarded and can in some instances even feel welcomed. Examples of this can be seen through narratives on the Schizophrenia Forum such as amusing and complimentary voices or visual hallucinations of 'cute vampires'. One post even stated:

> I found my 'psychosis' to be fun … I felt it was a magical experience, where I could use telepathy to communicate with others in the future and alike.

The sense of welcoming altered states of cognition is understandable if one's experience is not distressing. In some cases individuals can feel creatively liberated as William Blake is said to have been, actively embracing his 'madness' (Morris, 2006).

Boydell et al.'s (2006) study of first-episode psychosis found an individual avoidant strategy of ignoring and hiding early symptoms, with the persuasive influence of significant others in one's social network needed to seek help. As a NAMI (2011) survey demonstrated, individuals experiencing psychosis had differing perceptions to their families and friends about the presence of problems and the need for help. Seeking help however can be fraught with difficulties owing to the sense of trepidation about how others might respond. Dawson et al. (2013) confirm individuals with a first-episode psychosis often have a prolonged and complicated path to accessing appropriate treatment. The main barriers to seeking help were a fear of stigma and a reluctance to engage with agencies. A crisis experience and overt psychotic symptoms were the main promoters of active help-seeking, a stage where a person's ability to cope becomes more impacted upon and symptoms become more noticeable to others. There is concern over the length of time that symptoms go untreated and as McCann et al. (2011) state, easy access to first-episode psychosis services is critical in reducing the duration of untreated illness although primary caregivers can encounter difficulties accessing services. Their findings suggest that access should be influenced more by clinical need and less by caregivers' perseverance.

RECEIVING A DIAGNOSIS

Receiving a diagnosis can provoke a myriad of conflicting feelings from relief to terror (Pitt et al., 2009). Whilst it can help by 'naming the problem' it can also hinder by labelling the person and causing social exclusion. For some the receipt of a diagnosis will be influenced by what they understand about this diagnostic term, the level of distress and disruption currently experienced and the clarity of explanation given. Terms such as *psychosis* and *schizophrenia* are liable to conjure up a range of fears and fantasies and be viewed negatively. Schizophrenia, for example, is largely regarded as an unhelpful and restrictive diagnosis, applied too readily by practitioners. It carries an underlying message of chronic illness and a label which individuals carry with them for the rest of their lives.

> How would you feel if given a diagnosis with words such as 'schizophrenia' or 'psychosis' included?

Ken Steele (2002) recalled the look of worry, confusion and defeat on his parents' faces after being diagnosed with schizophrenia. He subsequently sought information from library books becoming increasingly unsettled and scared by what he read. Saks (2007) found her schizophrenia diagnosis damning and received it as if it were a death sentence. This brought about a significant shift in self-perception for her as pre-diagnosis, even though experiencing altered reality, she had not thought of herself as being ill. The shift from *mental well-health* to that of *mental ill-health* was also an impactful transition stage for Adamson (2013) with the feeling that this was now the beginning of the rest of her life. It was particularly distressing given the perceived stigmatising associations she linked with the film *Psycho* and Norman Bates.

These narratives illustrate the sense of trepidation felt with the prevailing negative connotations accessed through societal views or from the media. A posting on the Time to Change (2013a) website reflects this:

> Before this point, talking to anyone about my ailment was counter-productive. I'd say the word 'psychosis', which most were unfamiliar with (including myself), and then try to clarify with the word 'schizophrenia'. Not a particularly good idea, in hindsight. It turns out that using that word, thanks to the media, tends make people think you're a serial killer. That or, more bizarrely, that you share your body with an alter ego.

He goes on to express his envy towards individuals with depression or anorexia, conditions which he felt to a greater degree people understood.

This is shared by another narrative:

> I've got a diagnosis of [psychosis]. I don't feel comfortable describing myself in this way ... Psychotic is a terrible word which is associated in the public mind with extreme dangerousness ... Two of the most hurtful words in the dictionary: Schizophrenia and psychotic. Those two words can ruin your life.

Time to Change (2012a)

Being given a diagnostic label can be very hard given the powerful resonance that certain words have, although for some it may help to feel that one's chaotic and disparate symptoms have been given a name and that maybe now there is a sense of hope with treatment and support to follow. This is reflected by a personal narrative on the NHS Choices (2014b) website:

> The diagnosis was a relief. Yet all I knew about schizophrenia was what I'd read in the papers, that it was related to violence.

Likewise, a blogger writing on the Time to Change (2013b) website recounts:

> I have never been so relieved in all my life to know that there was something wrong and that people didn't actually hate me. I didn't care that I was now labelled with this illness just the feeling of relief that it wasn't all real was so great … I became a changed person after my diagnosis, I stopped keeping it all to myself and told my family all what I had been experiencing.

The experiences here illustrate the very varied and individual responses to receiving a diagnosis. What comes across strongly is the need for hope and affirmation that recovery is attainable to accompany any diagnosis delivery.

> What support or information do you feel people need at the point of diagnosis?

COMING TO TERMS/TELLING OTHERS

Coming to terms with a diagnosis of psychosis or schizophrenia can feel like a battle which can last for many years, with for some people resolution never being achieved.

Ken Steele (2002) recounts a strong process of denial concerning his mental health state which affected his whole family with his illness feeling like the 'elephant in the room'. This illustrates the difficulties in accommodating or accepting a person's illness. It can make it especially hard for people to open up about their problems and to get support from family and friends, seeing their difficulties as a weakness and something to feel ashamed of. This is illustrated by a narrative posted on the Time to Change website:

> The hardest issue I had to face was to tell my parents I was ill. I was a mess. Only certain friends knew that I was unwell, I felt that I couldn't tell the others something was wrong. I self-stigmatised myself, ashamed at how I could be so stupid and unable to do something. Here was a Cambridge graduate that could no longer cook pasta!
>
> Time to Change (2013c)

This provides a contrast between a person's current and former states, shared by Hill (1994, p. 28):

> It was a typical tragedy. Here was this graduate, who a few months earlier was the big success story of the family, turned into a poor shadow of his former self.

These narratives reflect a real change in thinking concerning the number of things which a person feels no longer able to do (or as perceived by others). There is a sense here of having transformed into a new self from wellness to illness. This transformation is largely viewed from a negative perspective with concerns about the thoughts and responses of others. Elyn Saks (2007) worried that opening up to her parents about her mental health difficulties would result in her being regarded as weak and a failure. She consequently concealed her schizophrenia diagnosis telling them instead about her co-existing depression and associated medication which felt easier. However, the sense of acceptance when people receive good responses can be a huge relief as reflected by the following narrative:

> I have recently started dating again. I found it hard to tell him [boyfriend] I had psychosis. It wasn't easy but I showed him who I was at first then after a few weeks I came out with it. He just took me for who I am, which was a relief. I've never had anyone take me for who I am in a relationship sense. They have always wanted me to be something I can't be, someone I'm not.
>
> Time to Change (2013b)

The decisions about what to reveal to others can be a continual dilemma with multiple possible occasions indicated. Pandya et al. (2011) found that individuals' disclosure about a schizophrenia diagnosis differed according to the type of social situation they were in, being more open with doctors, parents and friends than with employers or the police. There will be many instances in which a person feels unsure or unwilling to reveal their health status to others, feeling that it is just too difficult. It can also seem very hard to properly convey what one is experiencing to others as illustrated by Adamson (2013, p. 126) regarding her threatening, unseen (by others) presence:

> How do you convey that intensity and fear without people thinking you are a crazy? I do not tell people any more. Telling people just raises eyebrows.

It can feel very lonely having to keep difficulties to oneself as Schiller (1994) experienced feeling very separate from what she felt to be the billions of people making up the rest of humanity around her. The developing process of disconnectedness was also encountered by Ken Steele (2002) who in his autobiographical account documents feeling progressively more detached and alone. Social isolation is a significant problem for those experiencing mental health problems and can affect a person through a multitude of perspectives feeling psychically, psychological, socially and spiritually cut off and disengaged from the world around them.

Altered reality

This section examines what it is like to experience altered reality with manifestations such as hallucinations, delusional thoughts and disorganised thinking. The emotive experience can be threatening, terrifying and bewildering but also reassuring and seemingly 'normal'. It is important though to consider the impact upon a person's day-to-day life, employment, study and relationships.

HALLUCINATIONS

The term 'hallucination' can be defined as

> the apparent perception (usually by sight or hearing) of an external object when no such object is actually present.
>
> *Oxford English Dictionary* (2015)

Perhaps one of the most widely perceived symptoms concerning a psychotic disorder relates to hallucinations. Talking to oneself or responding to voices is commonly depicted within media products as an easily identifiable sign of 'madness', as shown, for example, by the chapter 'The Madness of Barty Crouch' in J.K. Rowling's (2000) *Harry Potter and the Goblet of Fire*. The reality though concerns an experience which for a large number of people can be completely 'normal' and encountered by individuals with no identifiable psychopathology (Romme and Escher, 1993). It can be experienced as supportive and reassuring, soothed, for example, by the voice of a significant person, who has perhaps died. Hallucinations can also torment and threaten individuals with risky or violent behaviours being influenced. Hallucinatory experience can come through any of the five senses:

1. Auditory (sound)
2. Visual (sight)
3. Tactile (touch)
4. Gustatory (taste)
5. Olfactory (smell)

The most prevalent form of hallucination is auditory, in particular voice hearing (Mental Health, 2006). There are numerous different manifestations with each person having their own individual experience. Voices can be intermittent or constant; supportive, benign or abusive; and heard as single voices or a series of voices. The experience of voice hearing in the general population ranges between 1% and 16% for adult non-clinical populations and 2% and 41% for healthy adolescent samples (Longden et al., 2012). Longden et al. (2012) describe voice hearing experiences in the context of psychotic disorders as dissociated or disowned components of the self that result from trauma, loss, or other interpersonal stressors.

Importantly, not all experiences are negative as a number of people describe feeling soothed and supported by their voices (Romme and Morris, 2009). These can be comforting and advising, appearing, for example, following a bereavement or trauma. Voices are initially helpful, forming the commencement of an integrative coping process and helping to boost self-esteem (Romme, 1989). Elisabeth Svanholmer (Svanholmer and Eyles, 2009) experiences a range of positive and negative voices, in particular Søren – an invisible friend who provides true friendship, support, understanding and respect. Similarly, a narrative from the Hearing Voices Network (2012) reflects:

> I have often found that one of my voices is more comforting and reassuring than those around me.

It can though commonly be distressing or threatening and for some people felt as a constant intrusion with little respite being found. John Frusciante, the ex-guitarist with the Red Hot Chili Peppers recalls:

> When I was 18, 19, 22, my brain was just clogged all the time – non-stop voices. I couldn't figure out what was going on. There was a lot of confusion inside me, this flood of voices, often contradicting each other, often telling me stuff that would happen in the future, and then it would happen, voices insulting me, telling me what to do.
>
> Hearing Voices Network (2012)

This illustrates some of the disruptiveness and distress caused to those involved including the imperative nature of voices telling a person what to do or think. Philip Hill (1994, p. 24) shares his experience of being instructed by his voices to seek out a woman that he had become infatuated with yet feeling desperate, hysterical and persecuted:

> I knelt down on the floor in a massive crying fit before banging my fists on the floor in sheer frustration. I then genuinely contemplated suicide.

These narratives reflect the difficulty in pursuing a 'normal' life. The distress and disruption to one's ability to cope and well-being are severely impacted upon when voices become threatening or abusive. The extent, duration and severity of the experience are also significant. Ken Steele (2002) was tormented for years by his voices, urging him to kill himself. It resulted in numerous suicide attempts and a growing isolation and separateness from others. The intensity can be such to prevent any real respite or escape from the experience as evidenced by Schiller's (1994) recollection. Whilst her voices started as a general background noise the intensity increased, becoming louder and more persistent. She had the sensation that like holding one's breath, keeping the voices at bay, could only be achieved for short periods of time. Further narrative examples can be found in Box 6.1.

How do you think you would you feel if you were experiencing voices?

Other types of hallucinatory experience are less common although can have an equally traumatising impact. Visual hallucinations, like other types, are experienced as *real* entities. In this case people, forms and shapes are perceived as present. Adamson (2013) relates her scary experience of 'seeing' men standing in her bedroom and her effective means of

Box 6.1 Hearing Voices Network (2015): Discussion forum

It's gotten to the point where my friends have screamed at me trying to get my attention but the voices were so loud I couldn't hear anything.

I can't formulate my words and I can't hear what people say, or concentrate on anything!

I have different types of voices and voice hearing and I have angels helping me ... companions that I hear and see.

dispelling the image by shining a torch or throwing things at them. A number of films provide the viewer with a glimpse at this experience with scenes in *Repulsion* (Gutowski and Polanski, 1985) or *A Beautiful Mind* (Grazer and Howard, 2001). This latter example about the Nobel Prize–winning mathematician John Nash includes a particularly potent scene interspersing what he sees and what other observers see. This provides a strong illustration of what the hallucinatory experience might feel like.

DELUSIONS/DISORGANISED THINKING

A delusion is

> a false belief based on an incorrect inference about reality that is firmly held despite the beliefs of almost everyone else, despite obvious proof to the contrary. The person holds a belief that is not ordinarily accepted by other members of the person's culture or subculture.
>
> American Psychiatric Association (2013)

Delusions are unshakeable beliefs which do not match up to the way other people see the world and tenuous evidence might be used to prove the way one sees things (Rethink Mental Illness, 2014). Different types of delusion can be seen in Box 6.2. Having thoughts and beliefs which are not shared by others engenders occasions for conflict. There may well be a strong dismissal from others who are unwilling to accept the validity of what they regard as fanciful or extreme. It is interesting to consider what resonance or significance delusional thoughts have for those concerned, even those which seem to be extremely bizarre and totally removed from reality. We might question the notion of what 'reality' is, especially if considering theoretical approaches such as Gestalt theory which

---

Box 6.2 Types of delusion

Persecutory (the person believes that they are being followed or is under surveillance, or that he/she is being made fun of, tricked, or treated very unfairly by others).

Delusions of reference (the person believes, for example, that things written in a newspaper or book, stated on television or expressed in a song are about them).

Grandiose delusions (the belief that a person has exceptional power, talent or worth, or is someone famous, i.e. God or some other type of deity).

Erotomanic delusions (the belief that a particular person, usually a celebrity or someone especially important, is romantically involved with or in love with them).

Somatic delusions (the belief that they have a medical condition or other physical problem or flaw).

Thought insertion, withdrawal, control, or broadcasting (the person believes that someone, often aliens, are putting (inserting) thoughts into his/her mind, removing or controlling his/her thoughts, or broadcasting them so that others can hear them, usually against his/her will).

Source: Schizophrenic, Types of delusion, 2015, Schizophrenic.com, accessed 12 June, 2015.

describes how each person constructs their own 'meaningful whole' or understanding of the world around them (Köhler, 1947). Davidson (1994) demonstrates how delusions can be viewed as stories that people tell about their lives and which can disclose lived experience. He further suggests that delusions may act as a regulatory mechanism helping people modulate the amount of change to which they will have to adapt in the context of significant life events.

Richard, a young man diagnosed with paranoid schizophrenia, relates the feeling that his thoughts occupy another layer of interaction with people and the world, as if there were two coexisting realities:

> If I'm listening to the radio, for instance, the rational part of me knows that the programme is being transmitted to lots of listeners and that it is a one-way form of communication. My delusional thinking, however, makes me believe that the radio can project what I say out loud to the people making the show and all the listeners.
>
> NHS Choices (2014c)

The words and language expressed within disorganised thinking can be dismissed as 'nonsensical', however can be very significant, as observed within the following narrative:

> Powerful whirlpools swirl around into a deep abyss. Stormy, frothy, violent waves crash down like loud explosions. These symbolize my strong emotions, and during this time, I hold onto myself with all my might and strength. I must survive.
>
> Molta (1997, p. 350)

This conveys a sense of experience with real poetic and symbolic meaning and can relate even when thinking becomes extremely and bizarrely distorted. As illustrated by Payne (1992, p. 726):

> My universe soon became populated [with alien beings]. The alien beings soon took over my body and removed me from it. They took me to a faraway place of beaches and sunlight and placed an Alien in my body to act like me. At this point I had the distinct impression that I did not really exist, because I could not make contact with my kidnapped self.

Whilst appearing totally abstract and fantastical, there are sub-themes being conveyed on a symbolic and emotional level. We can, for example, get a sense of the experience of feeling out of control as well as a sense of being disconnected and powerless. The sense of losing one's own volition and personal control can be very scary, as shown by Ruocchio (1991, p. 357):

> The worst thing possible is to be terrified of one's own mind, the very matter that controls all that we are and that we do and feel.

She describes the agony felt at not being able to think clearly and having a desperate sense of aloneness and separation from others. It is important to recognise and validate such expression in order to help individuals cope with what is occurring for them. The many available narrative accounts communicate much to us about lived experience. There is a need to find ways to tune in to and attend to the emotive content in what others are conveying. This can be seen in Hannah Green's (1964, p. 35) semi-autobiographical account of a 16-year-old girl's experience of schizophrenia:

> She saw the doctor's mouth moving, and imagined that it was spewing questions and accusations. She began to fall, going with Anterrabae through his fire-fragmented darkness into Yr. This time the fall was far. There was utter darkness for a long time and then a greyness, seen only in bands across the eye. ... The world intruded, but it was a shattered world and unrecognisable.

Whilst the words themselves are hard to understand, there is an undeniable sense of fear and helplessness being expressed, which is what can be related to. It is important to consider differences in interpretation between those experiencing disordered thinking and others around them. In a number of cases what is being expressed can be hard to comprehend by others whilst at the same time making perfect sense to the person experiencing thoughts.

VULNERABILITY (RISKS FROM SELF AND OTHERS)

The issue of vulnerability concerns personal risks of harm directed from others or from self. The risks to self are profound when experiencing a psychotic state. Contrary to stereotypical notions which perceive those with psychotic problems as posing a significant threat to others, the reality is that the greater risk concerns harm to self or exploitation by others. There is an excess mortality reported in patients with schizophrenia (Roy and Pompili, 2009) with suicide being one of the major contributors, especially in first-episode psychosis (Brown et al., 2000; Lopez-Morinigo et al., 2012). Perenyi and Forlano (2005) reviewed the identified risk factors for suicide in schizophrenia and found the most significant risk factors to include depression, the presence of positive symptoms and substance abuse. Fedyszyn et al. (2011) indicate that most suicide attempts tended to be impulsive (77.6%), triggered by interpersonal conflict or distress due to psychotic symptoms. Two-thirds involved self-poisoning, usually by overdose of prescribed medications, whilst most inpatient suicide attempts were by hanging or strangulation.

Suicidal thoughts can be influenced by a multitude of factors including altered cognition, delusional content, hallucinatory commands, depressed thinking and isolation. Indeed, in terms of depression, Reutfors et al. (2010) found that amongst patients with a clinical schizophrenia spectrum diagnosis, a mood disorder diagnosis increased the suicide risk more than threefold. A person's experience of altered cognition can result in many spheres in their life being impacted upon such as relationships, occupation, accommodation and lifestyle, developing periods of despair. The decision to attempt suicide can be followed by careful and meticulous planning or be something which is acted upon spontaneously. A person can also be harmed as a consequence of reckless behaviour, where there may be a sense of ambivalence about what might happen to them.

A number of people have documented the presence of suicidal thoughts in connection to hallucinatory experience. Adamson (2013) writes expressively about the meticulous preparation to kill herself, driven by her internal voices to act upon it. This can also, as Saks (2007) reflects, become more intense with the voices stepping up their demands, commanding her to kill herself. The risk is also exacerbated where a person, over time, engages in a series of suicide attempts. Ken Steele (2002, p. 179) recounts a steady succession of attempts coinciding with occasions when he was feeling more vulnerable, less supported and poorly occupied. At these times, he

> Became confused, disoriented and easy prey for the voices, which told me again and again what a terrible failure I was. I began drinking heavily and at all hours in a vain effort to drown the evil spirits inside me, demons that kept saying I was too old to live, too gross to live, too stupid to live.

Steele's (2002) biographical narrative is illustrative of the cyclical experience in which a person can function, in a sense gaining periods of respite but then awaiting the next wave of despair to wash over. Klonsky et al.'s (2012) study assessed hopelessness and attempted suicide at multiple points in time over a 10-year period in a first-admission cohort with psychosis. Their results suggest that even relatively modest levels of hopelessness appear to confer risk for suicide in psychotic disorders. This is extremely worrying given the multiple occasions with which one is liable to feeling hopeless. For Schiller (1994, p. 7), suicide attempts were a desperate means of coping with unresolved stress that built up. She regarded her mental health state (schizophrenia) as having

> snatched from me my tranquillity, sometimes my self-possession, and very nearly my life.

A feature for her though when surviving these attempts was the sense of having the lid blown off the seething cauldron of pressure which had built up internally. This left her for a short time feeling less distressed and with the voices lessened.

SELF-MEDICATION

Attempts to cope with distressing symptoms may involve self-medicating through the use of various substances including drugs, alcohol or nicotine. Substances of abuse help individuals relieve painful affects and control distressing emotions (Khantzian, 1997). Smoking rates in service users with schizophrenia are estimated to be two to four times the rate seen in the general population with stronger cigarettes favoured and more nicotine extracted from their cigarettes than other smokers (Kumari and Postma, 2005). Alcohol is widely abused amongst this group to alleviate symptoms as well as dealing with aspects such as boredom (Drake and Mueser, 2002). A further concerning issue with regard to drug use concerns the causative links between agents such as cannabis, cocaine and hallucinogens with psychosis (Dual Diagnosis, 2015). There is a selection of personal narratives about self-medication on the Schizophrenia discussion forum

Box 6.3 Schizophrenia discussion forum

I'm pretty sure I won't be able to quit [smoking] until my symptoms subside. If that ever happens.

[After smoking marihuana] I felt so dark and depressed; inside it's like your own soul had been removed from your body … I know it's not fun and a not a good idea to smoke when you are diagnosed, but I just really wanted the voices to go away.

Last night I got really high and had like 10 drinks in 2 hrs, figured it was better than the dark depression cloud that was looming over me. Paying for it today.

Now that I'm sober and looking back … I really have no idea why I thought drinking was as good as it was. Because I woke up in horrid shape every time … after a while … it took more and more to get drunk.

(see Box 6.3). These narratives display some of the feelings involved, whereby individuals attempt to balance their negative and positive feelings through the use of drugs, alcohol or tobacco. There are elements of desperation involved at wanting respite from symptoms. We can also read from such accounts a desire for personal control, to be able to deal with symptoms through one's own coping strategies and not remaining wholly reliant upon medical practitioners.

STIGMA

How do you expect stigmatising attitudes to affect individuals with psychosis/ schizophrenia?

People with mental health problems are amongst the most stigmatised groups in society (Bloch and Singh, 1997). Indeed, there is even a hierarchy of sorts which exist amongst mental health states with schizophrenia and psychoses commonly perceived to be at the far end of the spectrum. As Rose et al. (2011) highlight, negative discrimination can be connotatively very strong, with reports of humiliation and abuse encountered. The use of words is significant with a variety of associations conjured up, many of them inaccurate, upsetting and endurable. A blogger (Time to Change, 2013d) writes about her experience with schizophrenia and feels the quickest way to reduce the stigma would be to rename the condition. Indeed, perhaps years of sustained media and societal misrepresentation have left an indelible mark upon this condition. An interesting study in Korea (Kim et al., 2012) examined the change in term for schizophrenia from 'split-mind disorder' to 'attunement disorder'. The scores for prejudice regarding the danger posed by, and discrimination against, patients with schizophrenia were significantly higher in the group assigned split-mind disorder. This suggests that changing the name could reduce some of the prejudice and discrimination felt. The stigma is further reinforced by popular media products which convey notions of dangerousness, unpredictability and the age-old stereotype of *split personality*. These skewed and ill-informed examples have a significant impact upon people experiencing mental health problems as reflected by Ashley

Box 6.4 Stigma

When I'm told a person has schizophrenia,

I feel scared,

Anxious and apprehensive.

They frighten me and it's not a fear

That can be shared.

I would be considered prejudiced;

Not PC.

Yet schizophrenia is something that has happened to me.

...

If I told my friends about me

What would they say?

There would be talk

Would they want to stay away?

With constant voices on the brain,

One can crack under the strain

And act 'against the grain'.

Source: MacAskill, J., What is understanding, in: Carver, N. et al., eds., *Greater Goings On … (Than You Would Ever Guess …)*, Asylum Publishing, Sheffield, England, 2007, p. 51.

who reports feeling particularly bothered by the violent/aggressive stereotype and how he might be perceived by others (Choices in Recovery, 2011). This is also expressed very eloquently in the poem extract shown in Box 6.4.

Jenkins and Carpenter-Song (2009) investigated the subjective experience of stigma attached to schizophrenia-related disorders with 96% of participants reporting an awareness of stigma permeating their daily life. One aspect tied in with stigma awareness concerned being a 'person who regularly takes medication'. Individuals can also self-stigmatise, and Rusch et al. (2014) found young people experiencing early symptoms of psychosis self-labelling themselves as 'mentally ill' which was associated with reduced well-being. Gallo (1994) provides a personal illustration of this and how through self-stigmatisation individuals regarded selves as being relegated to the 'social garbage heap'. This resulted in becoming distanced from others and avoiding social contact, enduring years of self-torment and regarding selves very critically and dismissively. Another personal statement by Brundage (1983) sees stigma being the hardest aspect of the experienced difficulties to overcome. This can be related to feeling rejected or dismissed as, for example, highlighted by respondents in the INDIGO (2007) research study:

All my friends turned away from me when my neighbours found out about it, they said 'this lunatic has to be left alone'.

It is unsurprising to note the findings by Jenkins and Carpenter-Song (2008) highlighting the predicament of individuals with schizophrenia in recovery whose lives were still characterised as fraught with stigma. In considering the different types of stigma experienced, Cechnicki et al. (2011) found the most common experiences relating to the feeling of rejection by other people. This is significant especially with the acknowledgement that even the anticipation of discriminatory responses can lead some individuals to avoid participation in particular life areas thereby enhancing their sense of isolation (Farrelly et al., 2014). One aspect which seems particularly influential with regard to reducing stigma is the presence of role models. Saks (2007) makes a valid observation reflecting upon the comparative lack of role models, people with schizophrenia or psychosis who are living successful lives. Helen (Your Stories, 2012a) however points to individuals such as Rufus May and Ron Coleman, both having experienced psychotic difficulties yet contributing significantly towards clinical practice.

LOSS

A very strong and pervasive feeling for people affected with psychotic problems and their families concerns grief for lost opportunities. This is the sense of one's life remaining static or stalled whilst observing others getting married and starting a family, completing courses and training or gaining employment. BGW (2002, p. 746), a graduate student, recounts:

> For several years I was probably further away from reality than I have ever been. I felt certain that I would never again return to the stability and comforts of a sane mind. I was simply a vegetable. I could not read or write, watch TV, or even talk much of the time.

Molta (1997, p. 349) reflects:

> I have mourned the person I once was – someone who was so active and involved in life. Accepting my illness means accepting the fact I cannot do some things 'normal' people can do.

As well as tangible aspects which have been lost are the things which a person feels they were not able to achieve or have, in other words lost opportunities. This is vividly expressed by Lori Schiller (1994, p. 7):

> Along the way I have lost many things. the career I might have pursued, the husband I might have married, the children I might have had. During the years when my friends were marrying, having their babies and moving into the houses I once dreamed of living in, I have been behind locked doors, battling the Voices who took over my life without even asking my permission.

This sense of missing years, unfulfilled goals and lost opportunities is reflected by many narrative accounts. It reflects a grief reaction which respondents in Mauritz and van Meijel's (2009) related to feelings of loss concerning both internal and external aspects.

SECTION 2: EXPERIENCING SUPPORT

Interview narratives

Medication combined with counselling has been the most helpful.

I remember thinking on the ward that most of them don't give a monkey's, and they didn't. None of them spoke to me.

[My counsellor] is someone who clearly cares, she understands and treats me as a person ... I feel heard and listened to, not judged.

[Psychotherapy] calms down my thoughts to a place where I can cope with them. It slows things down and enables me to see things in a way that most people see the world.

I think it's really important for carers to recognise the validity of the experiences that people are having ... people are just experiencing different things to most other people but for them it will feel very real at the time.

I think mental health services tend to view people through a diagnosis more than the outside world does. Whereas the outside world might just say they're a bit wacky.

I've got some friends who have had psychosis and you feel an affinity, a different type of closeness that you don't get with other people.

Speaking to people who have had similar mental health experiences is helpful.

When troubled by psychosis or altered thinking, there are a variety of treatment interventions accessible. Some of these, highlighted earlier, include the innovative work of Marius Romme (1989) which inspired the development of the Hearing Voices Network. There are also a range of psychosocial interventions, vocational and community initiatives, social skills support and family education. Newer developing approaches include the Open Dialogue approach helping individuals and their families to cope with crisis situations and to engage in dialogue (Seikkula et al., 2011). More commonly accessed forms of support include psychotherapeutic interventions, medication, in-patient admission, family support, peer involvement and creative arts.

PSYCHOLOGICAL THERAPIES

How do you think people might be helped through psychotherapeutic interventions?

The National Institute for Health and Care Excellence (NICE, 2014) recommend that everyone with a diagnosis of schizophrenia or psychosis should be offered psychological therapy. Unfortunately, despite the high demand the vast majority of people still have no access to it or have to wait for a number of years. One of the core functions of psychotherapy is the connectedness that it affords those who may feel detached and separate from the world around them. Even when displaying extreme levels of distortion there is value in attempting to provide individuals with an *anchor* or steady base with which to ground themselves. Saks (2007, p. 232) experienced years of psychoanalytic work and greatly valued the security and containment it provided but was also struck by the importance of having her wildest thoughts validated:

> Kaplan had now seen my psychoses but wasn't scared by it.

This signifies an important moment concerning the fears and fantasises as to how one's psychotic thoughts might be responded to by others. A number of narrative accounts liken the psychotherapeutic process to a marathon or a battle. Indeed, what seems important is the stability and consistency which is provided allowing individuals to feel contained and secure. As Ruocchio (1989, p. 164) recounts:

> My therapist did not give in and after months of what felt like an intense war I was able to safely let him in, to feel him as real and to have true caring feelings about another person. I thought that letting my therapist in would destroy me but all it did was destroy a small part of my illness that kept me totally isolated from all other people.

This is immensely important and significant. Likewise McGrath (1984, p. 639) expresses:

> My therapist was not afraid to travel with me in my fearful times. She listens when I need to release some of the 'poisons' in my mind. She offers advice when I'm having difficulty with just daily living. She sees me as a human being.

The British Psychological Society (2014) support the need for talking therapies in that they help people make sense of their experiences, work out their meaning and identify what helps. They include a range of narratives in support of this intervention mode (see Box 6.5).

Psychological talking therapies are clearly valuable and help people to cope with troubling symptoms and feelings. They also help people hold and integrate fragmented or distorted thoughts whilst feeling accepted and heard. Persons recovering from schizophrenia often do not see themselves as possessing agency, social worth, or an integrated sense of themselves and their experiences (Lysaker et al., 2007). Therefore, it can be affirming and validating of individual self-worth and autonomy. It can also help people

---

Box 6.5 British Psychological Society: Psychotherapy (2014)

The difference made is amazing – it has really transformed my life … The only thing I regret is that I didn't have access to it sooner – it could have prevented a lot of suicide attempts and I wouldn't have felt so awful for so long.

Starting therapy was terrifying … But it soon became clear that Paul was not interested in my psychiatric label. And it was also clear he was prepared to address the issue of my voices without belittling them or treating them as weird … I feel that I am in control.

It enabled me to get in control of what was in my head. Everything is less chaotic and my mind is now freed up to do other things.

who have experienced years of difficulties. Grant et al. (2014) report upon the meaningful improvement in day-to-day life enabled through psychotherapeutic support given to Mary, a woman with schizophrenia. She had experienced 24 months without admission having previously been stuck in a cycle of repeated hospitalisations over two decades.

MEDICATION

A study by Jenkins et al. (2005) investigated the subjective experience of the process of improvement and recovery from the point of view of persons diagnosed with schizophrenia and schizo-affective disorders finding the subjective sense amongst the majority that taking medication plays a critical role in managing symptoms and avoiding hospitalisation. The different types of antipsychotic medication are 'typical' (older drugs) and 'atypical' (newer). Atypical medication can help with hallucinations, delusions, thought disorder, extreme mood swings and severe depression. They affect the action of neurotransmitters such as dopamine and serotonin (Royal College of Psychiatry, 2014).

Some of the newer 'atypical' antipsychotics include (BNF, 2015)

- Amisulpride
- Aripiprazole
- Clozapine
- Olanzapine
- Quetiapine
- Risperidone

There can be problems with medication compliance given the associated side effects (see Figure 6.2) which are borne out by a number of narrative accounts. The medication Schiller (1994) was taking left her feeling sick and hypersensitive to the sun, quickly getting burnt, whereas Adamson (2013) found the weight gain distressing. McGrath (1984) found medication helpful in relieving her mental stress but hated the dulling of

---

- Sleepiness and slowness
- Weight gain
- Sexual dysfunction
- Increased risk of diabetes
- Acute hypertension
- Parkinsonian side-effects, that is, stiffness of the limbs (high doses)
- Tardive dyskinesia (long-term use)
- Sensitivity to the sun
- Skin rashes
- Menstrual problems for women

How would you feel if you were presented with this list?

Figure 6.2 Side effects. (Adapted from Royal College of Psychiatry, Antipsychotics, 2014, http://www.rcpsych.ac.uk, accessed 17 January, 2015; National Institute for Mental Health, Schizophrenia, 2016, http://www.nimh.nih.gov/health/publications/schizophrenia-booklet-12-2015/nih-15-3517_151858.pdf, accessed 22 March, 2016.)

healthy emotions. She responded by stopping the medication as soon as the 'storm' subsided. There is a clear problem here which explains why non-compliance becomes an issue. Studies into antipsychotic medication adherence by patients with schizophrenia have shown a relatively low rate of compliance (Valenstein et al., 2004). Factors negatively influencing adherence include sexual dysfunction (Ucok et al., 2007), feelings of being used as experimental subjects (Rofail et al., 2009) and weight gain (Chiang et al., 2011). There are also factors to consider relating to what reliance upon medication means or symbolises for people. One dilemma concerns perspectives upon wellness and illness. Semar's (2000) phenomenological study highlighted the conflict participants felt in that in order to be normal one must take medication, yet to take medication to be normal means acknowledging the implication that one is not normal. This is reflected by Schiller (1994) who equated medication with being sick and so stopped taking it.

There are issues about getting the right balance or type of antipsychotic medication. In Dumas' (2000) study this meant finding one with tolerable side effects and that suppressed the illness enough for the individual to recover a sense of self. A problem and a common fear for a number of people is the perception that antipsychotic medication will make them 'zombified'. This was a particular problem with the older (typical) medication types with Parkinson's symptoms, stiffness in movements and sluggishness in thoughts (RCP, 2014). Whilst atypical medication is less likely to produce these effects they carry a heightened risk of producing diabetes, weight gain and sexual dysfunction (RCP, 2014). A study by Leslie and Rosenheck (2004) found 7.3% of those taking antipsychotic medication developing diabetes with the highest risk linked with clozapine and olanzapine. Song (2011) set out to identify the experience of antipsychotic medication interventions for women with schizophrenia identifying a number of problems. The recommendations were for the development of a safe and believable psychoactive drug considering the time of menstruation, pregnancy, childbirth, and child-raising.

For some people there are potential benefits from this type of intervention and for those with positive effects there is a higher incidence of compliance (Rettenbacher et al., 2004). Studies vary however and Keefe et al. (2007) found neurocognitive improvement associated with antipsychotic treatment in patients with schizophrenia to be small. Narrative accounts provide a variety of experiences. Stuart (NHS Choices, 2014b), a service user, feels that from taking medication his schizophrenic symptoms are totally under control. Other benefits can be seen within narratives from the British Psychological Society (2014) as illustrated in Box 6.6.

Box 6.6 British Psychological Society: Medication (2014)

With the new medication, I felt as sane as anyone, quite refreshed in mind, and wanted to go home immediately. As if by magic, the psychosis was finished.

The drug blocks out most of the damaging voices and delusions and keeps my mood stable.

Medication is a necessary evil as I have very little to fall back on otherwise. The medication stops psychotic symptoms, or has in the past.

I have to acknowledge the drug gave me my life back. Yes, I have tried to stop taking the drug to see if I no longer needed it and found the psychosis was still there.

It is clear that more is needed than just medication as a mode of symptom control. There are strong feelings though amongst those taking medication that it only deals with a part of the problem and that a holistic approach is needed (Murphy, 1997). The development of alternative treatment strategies is important for the large number of people with psychosis and schizophrenia who opt out of taking antipsychotic medication, or discontinue it because of adverse effects or lack of efficacy (NICE, 2014).

IN-PATIENT CARE

What do you envisage the experience of in-patient care to be like?

The type of environment individuals find themselves in when in need of extra help is important to their well-being and feeling of safety. In some cases this involves care in forensic units, a type of environment found in Hörberg et al.'s (2012) study to be perceived by patients as broadly non-caring. This is important to bear in mind when justifying and supporting the need for such units because of risk or containment needs. For those discharged into the community on community treatment orders, Light et al.'s (2014) research into lived experience found deficiencies in care with communication gaps and difficulty accessing services. The experience of in-patient treatment appears to be very variable regarded as both a 'safe' or terrifying place (NAMI, 2011). On the positive side hospital admission provides a place of safety, opportunities to stabilise medication and importantly, a renewal of hope. On the negative side is a high degree of frustration with the mental healthcare system, and decreased individual control. Schiller (1994) sums up the hospital experience (both positive and negative) as frightening, powerless, boring, secure and comforting.

Some people endure repeated admissions fluctuating between states of ill-health (relapse) and wellness. George and Howell's (1996) study of the rehospitalisation experience shows both positive and negative aspects. Each subsequent admission can be perceived as a marker of lost time with periods in hospital lasting for months or years. Recollection of these stays can appear hazy with people highlighting gaps in their memory, chunks of their life which to all intents and purposes have been erased. Ken Steele's (2002) narrative provides a clear illustration of this with one admission lasting for almost 2 years. He writes about various treatment interventions and recollections as if peering into a foggy scene. It is reminiscent of Charles Watkins' experience in Doris Lessing's (1971) *Briefing for a Descent into Hell* which charts the slow recovery to reality of a classics professor who has suffered a psychotic breakdown.

In-patient care can serve a confirming purpose of acknowledging one's problems and challenging the denial of what is occurring. This is reflected by Saks (2007, p. 62) for whom admission removed the pretence and confirmed that

I was a psychiatric patient, in a hospital for the mentally ill.

Time in hospital can provide stability and a chance to get one's life back on track. Paul (Your Stories, 2012b) experienced paranoia, voices and psychosis. Whilst in hospital he regained structure in his life, passed a number of GCSEs and subsequently set up his own print business. Herrig (1995) sees the time spent in hospital as being an opportunity to take stock, having space and time for reflection and thought. The time available though can also induce boredom and lack of activity (Schiller, 1994), with large portions of each day spent watching the clock or waiting for mealtimes (Steele, 2002).

One of the problems with being in hospital is the discontinuation from day-to-day life and loss of contact with family and friends. A blogger (Time to Change, 2013e) however on recovering from a psychotic episode found:

> Having visitors helped me keep my spirits up and believe I was going to go home soon … For me it meant the world. It meant normal life flowing into a place that was not normal at all. It meant relationships and connections that helped me build resilience.

The key elements here appear to be 'normality' and maintaining links with one's life outside of the hospital. The continuity factor is highly important as connections can easily become lost in the chaotic and fragmented experiences a person might encounter. This was very much Steele's (2002) experience and he found it very hard years later, when in recovery, regaining contact with his family.

CREATIVE ARTS

NICE (2014) recommend offering arts therapies to all people with psychosis or schizophrenia, particularly for the alleviation of negative symptoms. This enables people to experience themselves differently, develop new ways of relating to others and find ways to express selves. The communicative potential individuals have even though seemingly detached is well illustrated by the classic example concerning a woman, diagnosed with schizophrenia who rarely spoke yet created a piece of embroidery, rich with communicative meaning. This illustrated the connection she retained concerning the environment around her (Blakeman et al., 2013). It is important to look beyond a person's apparently incomprehensible communication or disengagement and utilise creative means for expression. In Sidhu and Eranti's (2010) study, the medium of art provided a safe creative space for service users to explore their thoughts and feelings, recognising the difficulty in verbal expression in early stages of psychosis. Alan Streets, a man diagnosed with schizophrenia was featured in a documentary, *My Name Is Alan and I Paint Pictures* (Boston, 2007). He expressed the importance that painting had for him in getting the negative, distorted thoughts out of his head, into his paints and then onto his brush and canvas. An important exhibition of art work was the *Seeing voices: Exploring psychotic experience through art and science*. This was held at Kings College London and provided a vivid variety of expressive pieces (Kings College, 2012).

Poetry provides another mode of communication, rich in expressive symbolism and meaning. Greek's (2010) study illustrated how counsellors can help with the trauma experienced during psychosis by reviewing hallucinations as personal and cultural symbols. This enables individuals to re-interpret their experiences, relieve anxiety and identify areas for improvement in their adaptation to the world around them. Music, another form of expression has proven to be significantly effective in suppressing and combating the symptoms of psychosis (DeBacker, 2008; Silverman, 2003). The range of creative modes can be extended further with positive results found with using drama (Casson, 2004), exercise (Ellis et al., 2007) and dance (Boydell, 2011).

FRIENDS AND FAMILY

A highly important factor in a person's recovery is the involvement and support of family and friends. Adamson (2013) regards the loving input of family and friends as providing a highly protective aspect, keeping her safe. The value can also be observed in a narrative posting on the Time to Change website:

> A core of friends visited and helped me extensively but some didn't ... One of the best things is just to be there for that person – just someone asking if I wanted to watch a film would have helped, making me feel a little more important.

Time to Change (2013c)

Another blogger (Time to Change, 2013f) relates how supportive friends helped her re-connect with the world. There were different responses from friends when she was most troubled by psychotic symptoms with some finding it hard to cope and be around her. Others though were able to listen to her, not defining her by her illness and waiting patiently day by day for her to get better. This mirrors some of the qualities and positive aspects identified earlier with regard to the psychotherapeutic process. People who are perceived to be constant, unfailingly supportive and accepting provide invaluable help. A blog posting (Time to Change, 2013g) praises her mum's help, someone who kept trying to reach the person (her daughter) beneath the mental health issues and

> Because she spoke to me, that part of me responded. She kept calling me gently back to who I am and back to my recovery.

This engagement from someone who cares is very impactful and was also experienced by a blogger in a text message received from his brother:

> Sorry that you're suffering. It's so tough isn't it. Thinking of you. You'll get there bruv x.

Time to Change (2014)

He recounts being deeply touched and surprised to receive such a heartfelt communication. What was vital though is that it also allowed him to feel safe, accepted and able to open up about his experience.

PEER SUPPORT

As with other mental health issues, a major support involves what can be gained (and given) to others who share experience of psychosis. There are a range of discussion forums including Schizophrenia, Hearing Voices Network, and Inter Voice within which individuals can share and discuss experience. Other essential resources for peer involvement include service user advocacy groups (Mind, Rethink Mental Illness) and health promotion/education initiatives (Time to Change). The discussion forums include people who are in desperate need of support and advice alongside those who have experienced similar aspects and are now in a position to help others. Opportunities to support others provide very important occasions to feel productive and help with recovery and the development of confidence and self-esteem (Brown, 2011). As previously noted, Elyn Saks (2007) complains about the comparative lack of positive role models concerning people with schizophrenia, people who have led successful and happy lives. She shows herself however to be an excellent role model, expressing her experience with eloquence and clarity providing real hope for others and helping to dispel a number of myths about schizophrenia. There are many other people promoting awareness and understanding of mental health experience through their involvement with educational institutions. A Time to Change (2012b) blogger experienced problems with psychosis and viewed the future bleakly as one involving medication, incarceration, and little hope of working or getting better. He subsequently found a role within a UK University as a Mental Wellbeing Advisor where his personal experience was used to help others, challenge stigma and discrimination and promote better attitudes to mental health. This experience is reflected through many related narratives illustrating the process of recovery and subsequent supporting of others. Though he once saw his diagnosis as a life sentence, Joshua now cites his schizophrenia as the difference in his life from seeing the world in black and white or seeing the world in colour. Joshua (Choices in Recovery, 2011) has a positive attitude about his experiences and is focused on and committed to helping others living with schizophrenia, working for the National Alliance on Mental Illness (NAMI), running peer-to-peer programs and sharing his story with other families.

SECTION 3: LIVING WELL

Interview narratives

I viewed the latest episode as a crisis in my identity where something needed to change. A phoenix – the psychosis is the fire and you go in and are reborn.

Your mind is going through something like you're developing … it jolts and suddenly goes off the tracks where it has to change.

[using personal experience] to support others makes me feel like I'm good at my job, that I'm special in some way. It's a big source of my self-esteem.

Listen, be kind and be yourself.

Having that experience [psychosis] was positive in terms of lifestyle. If I hadn't become acutely unwell I think I would have just continued doing the same sort of things I was doing … It's made me more aware of the importance of having a healthy balanced lifestyle where you are sleeping enough and taking care of yourself.

> To what degree do you feel it is possible to live well with psychosis/schizophrenia?

The World Mental Health Day on 10 October 2014 focused upon *Living with Schizophrenia*, which was concerned with showcasing examples of people living a health life with this condition. Initiatives such as this counteract stereotypical views which seem more concerned with deterioration and difficulties than of recovery and coping. An example of this in relation to postpartum psychosis is provided by a blogger who observes media reporting as being predominantly focused upon the risk posed to a baby's safety, with little attention given to the mother's recovery. She herself made a full recovery and importantly shares her story with medical students and health professionals (Time to Change, 2012c). In looking at what the term *recovery* means, participants in Forchuk et al.'s (2003) research described recovery from psychosis as a process that started with improvements in their thinking and feeling, and extended to a series of reconnections with their environment. These reconnections included staff and family. The focus of thought progressed from one's internal self to the world around them.

Eisenstadt et al.'s (2012) study regards recovery as the decrease or absence of psychotic symptoms, changes in social relationships, regaining autonomy and independence and restoration of self-reliance and trust in others. A core feature here is not looking for a state of *cure* but more one of *coping* as felt by Schiller (1994) when reaching a point of resolution and acceptance with her voices and finding ways to co-exist with them. The importance of finding resolution is illustrated by Payne's (1992) statement:

> This is not the life I thought I would live but it is a comfortable one filled with kind people.

As evidenced by McCarthy-Jones et al. (2013), the process of working through difficulties can be regarded as rebuilding and reforging with a degree of understanding and resilience being created. This was reflected by Adamson (2013) who recognised the positives in her overall experience, subsequently feeling as if she knew herself better. Interestingly, change even if involving a lessening of symptoms can be hard. When Ken Steele's (2002) voices of many years disappeared he recalled feeling more alone.

Recovery can be slow and progressive but something which can boost self-esteem and provide opportunities for resuming one's life:

> I am now doing really well after a lot of self-analysing and taking medication, I am now being able to go to work part time … I am so happy within myself and how I am now leading a normal life.
>
> Time to Change (2013b)

Recovery can mean reaching a point of feeling tougher and more resilient with newly developed personal resources (Brundage, 1983). A blogger sees her breakdown as having a silver lining. In recovery she commenced work as a human resource professional advocating a number of workplace wellness initiatives to prevent and raise awareness of mental health issues (Time to Change, 2012d). Another narrator relates the resumption of her life and relationships after 2 years of disruption stressing that it is possible to live one's life to the full even with mental health problems (Time to Change, 2013c). This positive message is shared by many other accounts.

A further aspect concerns the developing awareness of early warning signs of relapse (or signatures) which can help individuals attain a higher global functioning with fewer relapses (Birchwood et al., 2000; Sutton, 2004). This will differ from person to person with very individualised factors implied. There are however potential problems from raised insight with associated depression amongst some patients with schizophrenia (Browne et al., 1998). However, the importance here is in looking at what works best for each individuals and facilitating ways of feeling more in control.

Studies show that, over the long term (20 years), more than half of people with a diagnosis of schizophrenia experience clinical recovery (Slade, 2011). This recovery involves symptom remission, restoration of social functioning, and the development of social networks. Personal recovery involves the development of a life worth living. The orientation around personal recovery rather than clinical recovery is significant. In the Personal Recovery Framework (Slade, 2011), the individual experiences recovery through undertaking four recovery tasks:

1. Developing a positive identity outside of being a person with a mental illness
2. Developing a personally satisfactory meaning to frame the mental health experience (framed as a part of the person but not as the whole person)
3. Taking personal responsibility through self-management (responsible for own well-being, including seeking help when necessary)
4. Involving the acquisition of previous, modified or new valued social roles

A significant feature in recovery from psychosis is reaching a point of acceptance and making sense of one's experience. This is reflected by Rebecca who reached the point of recognising her mental health experience as something she had as opposed to defining who she was (Choices in Recovery, 2011). This marked a significant progression for her from an earlier point of feeling ashamed by her schizophrenia and unable to communicate her experience to family and friends. There is a point here of finding ways to accept one's difficulties. Schiller (1994) came to the realisation that she could not simply flip a switch (take the right pill or adjust thoughts in head) but needed to reach point of understanding her illness and learning to live with it. Likewise, Terry (Rethink Mental Illness, 2015) said that

> I've lived with paranoid schizophrenia for 12 years. For me, acceptance was the 'pass go' stage in my recovery journey – the first crucial step leading to real progress It involved admitting to myself that I do have a mental health problem and I need help.

There are some very important narratives here illustrating hope and resilience, but also seeing one's problems in a new light, as part of oneself yet not defining the whole self. As Nixon et al. (2010) found the experience of psychosis for some people is an important catalyst for spiritual and personally transformative growth. We are all different, and difference can be embraced and made the most of. At times support may be required but that in a sense applies to everybody whether experiencing mental health problems or not. People can live well with psychosis or altered cognition. Research by Hofer et al. (2004) with people with schizophrenia found more than half indicating that they were satisfied with life in general. As already shown, stigma is one of the harder aspects for people to cope with. Education about these conditions, continued health promotion, identification of positive role models, greater attention upon achievements and narratives about coping will help to improve the day-to-day experiences of those affected.

REFERENCES

Adamson, L. (2013). *The Voice Within: My Life with Schizophrenia*. Grosvenor House Publishing Limited: Guildford, England.

American Psychiatric Association (2013). *Diagnostic and Statistical Manual of Mental Disorders* (5th ed.). APA: Washington, DC.

Ballageer, T., Malla, A., Manchanda, R., Takhar, J. and Haricharan, R. (2005). Is adolescent-onset first-episode psychosis different from adult onset? *Journal of the American Academy of Child Adolescent Psychiatry*. 44(8), 782–789.

BGW (2002). Graduate student in peril: A first person account of schizophrenia. *Schizophrenia Bulletin*. 28(4), 745–755.

Birchwood, M., Spencer, E. and McGovern, D. (2000). Schizophrenia: Early warning signs. *Advances in Psychiatric Treatment*. 6(2), 93–101.

Blakeman, J.R., Samuelson, S.J. and McEvoy, K.N. (2013). Analysis of a silent voice: A qualitative inquiry of embroidery created by a patient with schizophrenia. *Journal of Psychosocial Nursing and Mental Health Services*. 51(6), 38–45.

Bloch, S. and Singh, B. (1997). *Understanding Troubled Minds: A Guide to Mental Illness and Its Treatment*. Melbourne University Press: Melbourne, Victoria, Australia.

Boston, J. (2007). *My Name is Alan and I Paint Pictures*. Raw Media Network, New York.

Boydell, K. (2011). Using performative art to communicate research. Dancing experiences of psychosis. *Canadian Theatre Review*. 146, 12–17.

Boydell, K., Gladstone, B. and Tiziana, V. (2006). Understanding help seeking delay in the prodrome to first episode psychosis: A secondary analysis of the perspectives of young people. *Psychiatric Rehabilitation Journal*. 30(1), 54–60.

British National Formulary (2015). BNF. https://www.medicinescomplete.com/mc/bnf/current/, accessed 19 November, 2015.

British Psychological Society (2014). Understanding psychosis and schizophrenia. http://www.bps.org.uk, accessed 3 May, 2015.

Brown, J.A. (2011). Talking about life after early psychosis: The impact on occupational performance. *Canadian Journal of Occupational Therapy*. 78(3), 156–163.

Brown, S., Barraclough, B. and Inskipp, H. (2000). Causes of the excess mortality of schizophrenia. A meta-analysis. *British Journal of Psychiatry*. 177(3), 212–217.

Browne, S., Garavan, J., Gervin, M., Roe, M., Larkin, C. and O'Callaghan, E. (1998). Quality of life in schizophrenia: Insight and subjective response to neuroleptics. *Journal of Nervous and Mental Disease*. 186, 74–78.

Brundage, B. (1983). First person account: What I wanted to know but was afraid to ask. *Schizophrenia Bulletin*. 9(4), 583–585.

Casson, J. (2004). *Drama, Psychotherapy and Psychosis: Dramatherapy and Psychodrama with People Who Hear Voices*. Routledge: London, UK.

Cechnicki, A., Angermeyer, M.C. and Bielanska, A. (2011). Anticipated and experienced stigma among people with schizophrenia: Its nature and correlates. *Social Psychiatry and Psychiatric Epidemiology*. 46(7), 643–650.

Chiang, Y.L., Klainin-Yobas, P., Ignacio, J. and Chng, C.M.L. (2011). The impact of antipsychotic side effects on attitudes towards medication in people with schizophrenia and related disorders. *Journal of Clinical Nursing*. 20(15–16), 2172–2182.

Choices in Recovery (2011). Living with schizophrenia: A call for hope and recovery. http://www.choicesinrecovery.com, accessed 18 October, 2014.

Cook, S. and Chambers, E. (2009). What helps and hinders people with psychotic conditions doing what they want in their daily lives. *The British Journal of Occupational Therapy*. 72(6), 238–248.

Davidson, L. (1994). Story telling and schizophrenia: Using narrative structure in phenomenological research. *The Humanistic Psychologist*. 21(2), 200–220.

Dawson, S., Jordan, Z. and Attard, M. (2013). Carers' experiences of seeking help for relatives with first-episode psychosis: A systematic review of qualitative evidence. *Database of Systematic Reviews and Implementation Reports*. 11(11), 183–361.

DeBacker, J. (2008). Music and psychosis. *Nordic Journal of Music Therapy*. 17(2), 89–104.

Drake, R.E. and Mueser, K.T. (2002). Co-occurring alcohol use disorder and schizophrenia. *National Institute on Alcohol Abuse and Alcoholism*. 26(2), 99–102.

Dual Diagnosis (2015). What is stimulant-induced psychosis. http://www.dualdiagnosis.org/, accessed 6 June, 2015.

Dumas, R.E. (2000). The lived experience of taking neuroleptic medication by persons with schizophrenia. Doctoral dissertation. University of Arizona: Tucson, AZ.

Eisenstadt, P., Monteiro, V.B., Diniz, M.J. and Chaves, A.C. (2012). Experience of recovery from a first-episode psychosis. *Early Intervention in Psychiatry*. 6(4), 476–480.

Ellis, N., Crone, D., Davey, R. and Grogan, S. (2007). Exercise interventions as an adjunct therapy for psychosis: A critical review. *British Journal of Clinical Psychology*. 46(1), 95–111.

Farrelly, B. and Farrelly, P. (2000). *Me, Myself and Irene*. Twentieth Century Fox Film Corporation: United States.

Farrelly, S., Clement, S., Gabbidon, J., Jeffery, D., Dockery, L., Lassman, F. et al. (2014). Anticipated and experienced discrimination amongst people with schizophrenia, bipolar disorder and major depressive disorder: A cross sectional study. *BMC Psychiatry*. 14(1), 157.

Fedyszyn, I.E., Harris, M.G., Robinson, J., Edwards, J. and Paxton, S.J. (2011). Characteristics of suicide attempts in young people undergoing treatment for first episode psychosis. *Australian and New Zealand Journal of Psychiatry*. 45(10), 838–845.

Forchuk, C., Jewell, J., Tweedell, D. and Steinnagel, L. (2003). Reconnecting: The client experience of recovery from psychosis. *Perspectives in Psychiatric Care*. 39(4), 141–150.

Gallo, K. (1994). First person account: Self-stigmatization. *Schizophrenia Bulletin*. 20(2), 407–411.

George, R.D. and Howell, C.C. (1996). Clients with schizophrenia and their caregivers' perceptions of frequent psychiatric rehospitalizations. *Issues in Mental Health Nursing.* 17(6), 573–588.

Grant, P.M., Reisweber, J., Luther, L., Brinen, A.P. and Beck, A.T. (2014). Successfully breaking a 20-year cycle of hospitalizations with recovery-oriented cognitive therapy for schizophrenia. *Psychological Services.* 11(2), 125–133.

Grazer, B. and Howard, R. (2001). *A Beautiful Mind.* Universal Pictures: United States.

Greek, M.T. (2010). How a series of hallucinations tells a symbolic story. *Schizophrenia Bulletin.* 36(6), 1033–1065.

Green, H. (1964). *I Never Promised You a Rose Garden.* Signet: New York.

Gutowski, G. and Polanski, R. (1985). *Repulsion.* Compton Films: UK.

Hearing Voices Network (2012). Discussion forum. http://www.hearing-voices.org/, accessed 13 June, 2015.

Hearing Voices Network (2015). Discussion forum. http://www.hearing-voices.org/, accessed 13 June, 2015.

Herrig, E. (1995). First person account: A personal experience. *Schizophrenia Bulletin.* 21(2), 339–342.

Hill, P. (1994). *Femme Fatale: A Personal Experience of Schizophrenia.* Autobiographical Publications: Birmingham, England.

Hofer, A., Kemmler, G., Eder, U., Edlinger, M., Hummer, M. and Fleischhacker, W. (2004). Quality of life in schizophrenia: The impact of psychopathology, attitude toward medication, and side effects. *Journal of Clinical Psychiatry.* 65(7), 932–939.

Hörberg, U., Sjögren, R. and Dahlberg, J. (2012). To be strategically struggling against resignation: The lived experience of being cared for in forensic psychiatric care. *Issues in Mental Health Nursing.* 33(11), 743–751.

INDIGO (2007). Towards mental health. http://www.kcl.ac.uk, accessed 22 July, 2015.

Inter Voice. (2015). Online discussion forum. http://www.intervoiceonline.org/, accessed 23 July, 2015.

Jenkins, J.H. and Carpenter-Song, E. (2008). Stigma despite recovery: Strategies for living in the aftermath of psychosis. *Medical Anthropology Quarterly.* 22(4), 381–409.

Jenkins, J.H. and Carpenter-Song, E. (2009). Awareness of stigma among persons with schizophrenia: Marking the contexts of lived experience. *The Journal of Nervous and Mental Disease.* 197(7), 520–529.

Jenkins, J.H., Strauss, M.E., Carpenter, E.A., Miller, D., Floersch, J. and Sajatovic, M. (2005). Subjective experience of recovery from schizophrenia-related disorders and atypical antipsychotics. *International Journal of Social Psychiatry.* 51(3), 211–217.

Keefe, R., Bilder, R., Davis, S., Harvey, P., Palmer, B., Gold, J. et al. (2007). Neurocognitive effects of antipsychotic medications in patients with chronic schizophrenia in the CATIE trial. *Archives of General Psychiatry.* 64(6), 633–647.

Khantzian, E.J. (1997). The self-medication hypothesis of substance use disorders: A reconsideration and recent applications. *Harvard Review of Psychiatry.* 4(5), 231–244.

Kim, S.W., Jang, J.E., Kim, J.M., Shin, I.S., Ban, D.H., Choi, B. et al. (2012). Comparison of stigma according to the term used for schizophrenia: Split-mind disorder vs attunement disorder. *Journal of the Korean Neuropsychiatric Association.* 51(4), 210–217.

Kings College (2012). Seeing voices: Exploring psychotic experience through art and science. http://www.kcl.ac.uk/artshums/ahri/eventrecords/SeeingVoices.aspx, accessed 1 April, 2015.

Klonsky, E., Kotov, R., Bakst, S., Rabinowitz, J. and Bromet, E.J. (2012). Hopelessness as a predictor of attempted suicide among first admission patients with psychosis: A 10-year cohort study. *Suicide & Life-Threatening Behavior.* 42(1), 1–10.

Köhler, W. (1947). *Gestalt Psychology: The Definitive Statement of the Gestalt Theory.* Liveright Publishing Corporation: New York.

Kumari, V. and Postma, P. (2005). Nicotine use in schizophrenia: The self medication hypotheses. *Neuroscience & Biobehavioral Reviews.* 29(6), 1021–1034.

Leslie, D. and Rosenheck, R. (2004). Incidence of newly diagnosed diabetes attributable to atypical antipsychotic medications. *The Journal of American Psychiatry.* 161(9), 1709–1711.

Lessing, D. (1971). *Briefing for a Descent into Hell.* Panther: Suffolk, England.

Light, E.M., Robertson, M.D., Boyce, P., Carney, T., Rosen, A., Cleary, M. et al. (2014). The lived experience of involuntary community treatment: A qualitative study of mental health consumers and carers. *Australasian Psychiatry.* 22(4), 345–351.

Lloyd, T., Dazzan, P., Dean, K., Park, S., Fearon, P., Doody, G.A. et al. (2008). Minor physical anomalies in patients with first-episode psychosis: Their frequency and diagnostic specificity. *Psychological Medicine.* 38(1), 71–77.

Longden, E., Madill, A. and Waterman, M.G. (2012). Dissociation, trauma, and the role of lived experience: Toward a new conceptualization of voice hearing. *Psychological Bulletin.* 138(1), 28–76.

Lopez-Morinigo, J.D., Ramos-Rios, R., David, A.S. and Dutta, R. (2012). Insight in schizophrenia and risk of suicide: A systematic update. *Comprehensive Psychiatry.* 53(4), 313–322.

Lysaker, P., Buck, K. and Roe, D. (2007). Psychotherapy and recovery in schizophrenia: A proposal of key elements for an integrative psychotherapy attuned to narrative in schizophrenia. *Psychological Services.* 4(1), 28–37.

MacAskill, J. (2007). What is understanding. In N. Carver, J. Morrison, N. Clibbens and T. Simpson (Eds.), *Greater Goings On … (Than You Would Ever Guess …)* (p. 51). Asylum Publishing: Sheffield, England.

Mauritz, M. and van Meijel, B. (2009). Loss and grief in patients with schizophrenia: On living in another world. *Archives of Psychiatric Nursing.* 23(3), 251–260.

McCann, T.V., Lubman, D.I. and Clark, E. (2011). First-time primary caregivers' experience accessing first-episode psychosis services. *Early Intervention in Psychiatry.* 5(2), 156–162.

McCarthy-Jones, S., Marriott, M., Knowles, R., Rowse, G. and Thompson, A.R. (2013). What is psychosis? A meta-synthesis of inductive qualitative studies exploring the experience of psychosis. *Psychosis: Psychological, Social and Integrative Approaches.* 5(1), 1–16.

McGrath, M. (1984). First person account: Where did I go? *Schizophrenia Bulletin.* 10(4), 638–640.

Mental Health (2006). Symptoms of schizophrenia. http://psychcentral.com, accessed 16 April, 2015.

Molta, V. (1997). First person account: Living with mental illness. *Schizophrenia Bulletin.* 23(2), 349–351.

Morrall, P. (2000). *Madness and Murder*. Whurr: London, UK.

Morris, G. (2006). *Mental Health Issues and the Media*. Routledge: London, UK.

Murphy, M. (1997). First person account: Meaning of psychoses. *Schizophrenia Bulletin*. 23(3), 541–543.

NAMI (2011). First episode psychosis. http://www2.nami.org, accessed 18 March, 2015.

National Institute for Mental Health (2016). Schizophrenia. http://www.nimh.nih.gov/health/publications/schizophrenia-booklet-12-2015/nih-15-3517_151858.pdf, accessed 22 March, 2016.

NHS Choices (2014a). Schizophrenia. http://www.nhs.uk, accessed 19 January, 2015.

NHS Choices (2014b). Schizophrenia: Stuart's story. http://www.nhs.uk, accessed 19 January, 2015.

NHS Choices (2014c). Schizophrenia: Richard's story. http://www.nhs.uk, accessed 19 January, 2015.

NICE (2014). Psychosis and schizophrenia in adults: Treatment and management. http://www.nice.org.uk, accessed 22 February, 2015.

NIMH (2015). Schizophrenia. http://www.nimh.nih.gov, accessed 16 August, 2015.

Nixon, G., Hagen, B. and Peters, T. (2010). Psychosis and transformation: A phenomenological inquiry. *International Journal of Mental Health and Addiction*. 8(4), 527–544.

Oxford English Dictionary (2015). Hallucination. http://www.oed.com/, accessed 14 September, 2015.

Pandya, A., Bresee, C., Duckworth, K., Gay, K. and Fitzpatrick, M. (2011). Perceived impact of the disclosure of a schizophrenia diagnosis. *Community Mental Health Journal*. 47(6), 613–621.

Payne, R. (1992). First person account: My schizophrenia. *Schizophrenia Bulletin*. 18(4), 725–727.

Perenyi, A. and Forlano, R. (2005). Suicide in schizophrenia. *Neuropsychopharmacologia Hungarica*. 7(3), 107–117.

Pitt, L., Kilbride, M., Welford, M., Nothard, S. and Morrison, A.P. (2009). Impact of a diagnosis of psychosis: User-led qualitative study. *Psychiatric Bulletin*. 33(11), 419–423.

Rethink Mental Illness (2014). Schizophrenia. https://www.rethink.org, accessed 19 January, 2015.

Rethink Mental Illness (2015). Terry's recovery story. http://www.rethink.org, accessed 2 August, 2015.

Rettenbacher, M.A., Hofer, A., Eder, U., Hummer, M., Kemmler, G., Weiss, E.M. and Fleischhacker, W. (2004). Compliance in schizophrenia: Psychopathology, side effects, and patients' attitudes toward the illness and medication. *Journal of Clinical Psychiatry*. 65(9), 1211–1218.

Reutfors, J., Bahmanyar, S., Jonsson, E.G., Ekbom, A., Nordstrom, P., Brandt, L. and Osby, U. (2010). Diagnostic profile and suicide risk in schizophrenia spectrum disorder. *Schizophrenia Research*. 123(2–3), 251–256.

Rofail, D., Heelis, R. and Gournay, K. (2009). Results of a thematic analysis to explore the experiences of patients with schizophrenia taking antipsychotic medication. *Clinical Therapeutics*. 31(1), 1488–1496.

Romme, M. (1989). Hearing voices. *Schizophrenia Bulletin*. 15(2), 209–216.

Romme, M. and Escher, S. (1993). *Accepting Voices*. Mind Publications: London, UK.

Romme, M. and Morris, M. (2009). Introduction. In M. Romme, S. Escher, J. Dillon, D. Corstens and M. Morris (Eds.), *Living with Voices* (pp. 1–6). PCCS Books: Ross-on-Wye, England.

Rose, D., Willis, R., Brohan, E., Sartorius, N., Villares, C., Wahlbeck, K. and Thornicroft, G. (2011). Reported stigma and discrimination by people with a diagnosis of schizophrenia. *Epidemiology and Psychiatric Sciences*. 20(2), 193–204.

Rowling, J.K. (2000). *Harry Potter and the Goblet of Fire*. Scholastic Inc.: New York.

Roy, A. and Pompili, M. (2009). Management of schizophrenia with suicide risk. *Psychiatric Clinics of North America*. 32(4), 863–883.

Royal College of Psychiatry (2014). Antipsychotics. http://www.rcpsych.ac.uk, accessed 17 January, 2015.

Ruocchio, P. (1989). First person account: Fighting the fight – The schizophrenic's nightmare. *Schizophrenia Bulletin*. 15(1), 163–166.

Ruocchio, P. (1991). First person account: The schizophrenic inside. *Schizophrenia Bulletin*. 17(2), 357–360.

Rusch, N., Corrigan, P.W., Heekeren, K., Theodoridou, A., Dvorsky, D., Metzler, S. et al. (2014). Well-being among persons at risk of psychosis: The role of self-labeling, shame, and stigma stress. *Psychiatric Services*. 65(4), 483–489.

Saks, E. (2007). *The Centre Cannot Hold – A Memoir of My Schizophrenia*. Virago: London, UK.

Schiller, L. (1994). *The Quiet Room*. Warner Books: New York.

Schizophrenia Forum. (2015). Forum. http://forum.schizophrenia.com/, accessed 23 July, 2015.

Seikkula, J., Alakare, B. and Aaltonen, J. (2011). The Comprehensive Open-Dialogue Approach in Western Lapland: II. Long-term stability of acute psychosis outcomes in advanced community care. *Psychosis: Psychological, Social and Integrative Approaches*. 3(3), 192–204.

Semar, D. (2000). Making my own acquaintance: A phenomenological study of taking antipsychotic medication for schizophrenia. Doctoral dissertation. University of Connecticut, Storrs, CT.

Sidhu, R. and Eranti, S.V. (November 2010). Role of art therapy in early intervention. Early intervention in psychiatry. Paper presented at *Seventh International Conference on Early Psychosis*, Amsterdam, the Netherlands.

Silverman, M.J. (2003). The influence of music on the symptoms of psychosis: A meta-analysis. *Journal of Music Therapy*. 40(1), 27–40.

Slade, M. (2011). The journey of recovery: Moving through tokenism to meaningful change. *Psychiatrische Praxis*. 38, s01.

Song, E.J. (2011). The lived experience of the women with schizophrenia taking antipsychotic medication. *Journal of Korean Academy of Nursing*. 41(3), 382–392.

Steele, K. (2002). *The Day the Voices Stopped*. Basic Books: New York.

Sutton, D.L. (2004). Relapse signatures and insight: Implications for CPNs. *Journal of Psychiatric and Mental Health Nursing*. 11(5), 569–574.

Svanholmer, E. and Eyles, T. (2009). Elisabeth Svanholmer. In M. Romme, S. Escher, J. Dillon, D. Corstens and M. Morri (Eds.), *Living with Voices* (pp. 147–152). PCCS Books: Ross-on-Wye, England.

Time to Change (2012a). Personal narrative. http://www.time-to-change.org.uk, accessed 18 November, 2014.

Time to Change (2012b). Personal narrative. http://www.time-to-change.org.uk, accessed 18 November, 2014.

Time to Change (2012c). Personal narrative. http://www.time-to-change.org.uk, accessed 18 November, 2014.

Time to Change (2012d). Personal narrative. http://www.time-to-change.org.uk, accessed 18 November, 2014.

Time to Change (2013a). Personal narrative. http://www.time-to-change.org.uk, accessed 16 November, 2014.

Time to Change (2013b). Personal narrative. http://www.time-to-change.org.uk, accessed 16 November, 2014.

Time to Change (2013c). Personal narrative. http://www.time-to-change.org.uk, accessed 16 November, 2014.

Time to Change (2013d). Personal narrative. http://www.time-to-change.org.uk, accessed 16 November, 2014.

Time to Change (2013e). Personal narrative. http://www.time-to-change.org.uk, accessed 16 November, 2014.

Time to Change (2013f). Personal narrative. http://www.time-to-change.org.uk, accessed 16 November, 2014.

Time to Change (2013g). Personal narrative. http://www.time-to-change.org.uk, accessed 16 November, 2014.

Time to Change (2014). Personal narrative. http://www.time-to-change.org.uk, accessed 16 November, 2014.

Ucok, A., Incesu, C., Aker, T. and Erkoc, S. (2007). Sexual dysfunction in patients with schizophrenia on antipsychotic medication. *European Psychiatry*. 22(5), 328–333.

Valenstein, M., Blow, F., Copeland, L., McCarthy, J., Zeber, J., Gillon, L. et al. (2004). Poor antipsychotic adherence among patients with schizophrenia: Medication and patient factors. *Schizophrenia Bulletin*. 30(2), 255–264.

Your Stories (2012a). Helen Williams. http://www.leedsandyorkpft.nhs.uk, accessed 28 June, 2015.

Your Stories (2012b). Paul Frazer. http://www.leedsandyorkpft.nhs.uk, accessed 28 June, 2015.

'Patching over the holes'
Living with impaired cognition

INTRODUCTION

The themes covered in this chapter reflect some of the thoughts and feelings relating to an ongoing deterioration in one's capabilities and cognition due to the presence of dementia. It is a condition which is largely misunderstood or commonly viewed from a predominantly negative perspective. Diagnosis is prone to being regarded as a 'hopeless' scenario with fears and attention predominantly placed upon perceived and experienced difficulties. The nature of problems experienced will be wide ranging and will differ significantly from person to person. The decrease in a person's cognitive ability impacts across all holistic dimensions with depression, loss, anxiety, isolation, dependence, mobility and communication all featuring strongly. Supportive interventions for people with dementia are very variable, ranging from effective and helpful approaches to those which are depersonalising, fostering of dependency or simply abusive. In order to better contextualise these issues the focus within this chapter is upon the internal experiences of the condition of dementia and the types of support and help available. A point of note restricting the accessing of personal narratives relates to the general decrease in a person's communicative ability. This can be matched by our decreasing capacity or inclination to understand what a person with dementia might be conveying. This work strives to stay with what is being expressed and acknowledge and appreciate more of the personal journey with dementia.

SECTION 1: EXPERIENCING DEMENTIA

Interview narratives

One particular incident, I couldn't find my purse. I know it sounds ridiculous, I had bought some pastry and had put the pastry into my handbag and my purse into the freezer.

Until you get the diagnosis you feel you're going crazy ... but once you know it helps.

When I found out [I had Alzheimer's] I cried me eyes out. But I'm doing alright now.

People say to me what did you do when so and so happened. Well how the bloody hell should I know. It happened so long ago and it's gone.

It is so frustrating when you want to say something but you can't get it across.

> I say I am going to vacuum round and he [my husband] says no you're not I'll do that and I say to him look you've got to let me do what I still can, while I can .... He don't let me iron although I don't particularly mind that because I don't like ironing.
>
> A lot of people are ignorant about dementia and Alzheimer's. People think you're mad which isn't very nice. It isn't very nice when you hear people say oh she's mad, her. That's that woman who's got that disease.

Briefly consider what image the term 'person with dementia' conjures up for with regard to a person's

- Appearance
- Behaviour
- Capabilities

The term 'person with dementia' generally conjures up thoughts and images of frail elderly people in the later stages of this condition, detached from their former lives, uncommunicative, sitting passively within care homes and dependent upon others for their care needs. This perhaps is the stereotypical view of a person at the stage where decline has greatly hampered and impeded their abilities. It does not accurately represent the millions of people worldwide with this condition who continue to function effectively, maintaining a positive quality of life. This skewed perception projects people to an advanced stage of their condition, to a point where they are unable to self-care and requiring full-time residential assistance. The fact that diagnoses are now being made at earlier stages, when symptoms are less discernible to other people, needs recognising. This is a point within the dementia journey where many people are still productive, actively engaged in work and leisure pursuits, able to drive and conduct busy social lives. Getting inside the dementia experience means understanding who people are, how their lives are being affected and essentially what they are still able to do. This encompasses a holistic perspective which not only appreciates the organic changes taking place in a person's brain, but also for instance how a person might be affected by the lowered expectations of others, co-existing states of depression and anxiety, and reduced social functioning. It is essential that we take stock of the wider picture and properly contextualise what a person's experience means to them along with the multitude of influencing factors, both internal and external.

DEMENTIA STATISTICS

Globally, the number of people living with dementia worldwide was estimated in 2015 to be 47.5 million, a figure projected to increase to 75.6 million by 2030 (WHO, 2015). In the United Kingdom numbers are similarly increasing estimated to rise from the current figure of 850,000 to 1 million by 2025 and 2 million by 2051 (Alzheimer's Society, 2014a). These are alarming statistics linked to a number of aspects such as an aging population and lifestyle factors.

TYPES OF DEMENTIA

It is worth initially pointing out that the terms 'Alzheimer's' and 'dementia' are often used synonymously with little understanding of the range of conditions which fall under the umbrella term *dementia*. The Alzheimer's Society provides a number of factsheets concerning the different types of dementia. Extracts from this information is combined here with related personal narratives from individuals living with these varied types of dementia.

Alzheimer's disease is the most common type of dementia, caused by the development of protein deposits ('plaques' and 'tangles') and a shortage of important chemicals involved with the transmission of messages within the brain. It is a progressively developing condition causing problems with memory, finding the right words, confusion, mood swings, withdrawal, and difficulties carrying out everyday activities. Chris Roberts (2014a), a 53-year-old man with early-onset Alzheimer's, details the distressing feelings associated with his deteriorating independence:

> It starts in the morning, I wake up and sometimes can't remember what comes next, I lie there racking my brain, trying to remember, sometimes I shout my wife and she has to explain and hint about getting up, gentle reminders to shower, to dress, to put on clean clothes. Otherwise without these reminders I wouldn't remember to shower and dress in clean clothes. I forget to eat, I forget what I've actually eaten … If, when leaving a room [the door is shut] I CANT GET OUT! The first time this happened I just sat down and cried.

This short narrative encapsulates a wide range of feelings including helplessness, frustration, distress and anger. It highlights some of the despair that can be felt concerning the process of enforced dependency.

Vascular dementia is the second most common form of dementia caused by problems in the supply of blood to the brain, for example, following a stroke. It often follows a 'stepped' progression, with symptoms remaining at a constant level for a while and then suddenly deteriorating. People with vascular dementia may experience problems with thinking, concentration, memory, communication and confusion. Other symptoms include misperceptions, behaviour changes, hallucinations and mobility. Functioning can periodically deteriorate very quickly leaving those affected and others close to them bewildered and frightened by the rapid change. These aspects can have a significant impact upon individuals' daily lives, and as Trevor Jarvis (Dementia Friends, 2012) reflected:

> It goes without saying that dementia has changed my life … One such occasion recently was when I was in my local bank trying to deposit some money. Unbeknown to me I was doing something wrong – pressing the wrong button or entering the wrong number, I'm still not sure. The response of the cashier was to point me towards a sign. But as my dementia can affect my ability to read, this was of very little use to me. Obviously confused, I received no more help from either the staff or the other customers in the bank.

This was related to *Dementia Friends*, an initiative set up by the Alzheimer's Society to make people's everyday lives easier.

Dementia with Lewy bodies (DLB) shares symptoms with Alzheimer's and Parkinson's. Lewy bodies are tiny deposits of protein in nerve cells which affect chemical messengers in the brain. Over time, there is progressive death of nerve cells and loss of brain tissue. Symptoms include impaired movement (i.e. rigidity and stooped posture), risk of falls, impaired attention and alertness, perceptual difficulties, planning and organising. Other symptoms include memory problems, hallucinations, sleep disorders and blank facial expression. Silverfox (2014a) compares his experience of living with DLB to having had too much to drink with effects such as slurred speech, drooling and feeling confused:

> Today, I see the world around me at a distance. My brain is responding very slowly. My vision is fuzzy. And my body movements are slow and clumsy ... Right now, I feel like I have been drinking, steady, for a while! Things look distant to me. I am tired, lethargic, and disoriented.

This narrative illustrates the difficulty in functioning and how withdrawal from daily activities can be influenced.

Fronto-temporal dementia (FTD) (Pick's disease or frontal lobe dementia) is one of the less common forms of dementia and is caused by damage to the frontal lobes. Symptoms include changes in personality and behaviour; difficulties with language, planning, organising or making decisions; and loss of inhibitions, interest, motivation, sympathy and empathy. There may be repetitive, compulsive or ritualised behaviours as well changes. Howard Glick (2014) relates:

> FTD is a very lonely disease. Day in, day out you don't recognize yourself and are estranged from those around you. No worse feeling in the world than knowing you love your kids, but don't feel comfortable around them ... I don't keep food at home because I eat spoiled food, food left around and even eat it off the floor. I don't like eating out because my behaviour around people gets me in trouble.

This provides a terrifying insight of Glick's internal world and the increasing sense of separateness and isolation which can develop through FTD.

Other dementias include Korsakoff's syndrome (associated with heavy drinking over a long period), HIV-related cognitive impairment, particularly in the later stages of a person's illness and Creutzfeldt–Jakob disease which is caused by infectious agents. There are many other rarer causes of dementia, including corticobasal degeneration, Huntington's disease, multiple sclerosis, Niemann–Pick disease type C, normal pressure hydrocephalus, Parkinson's disease, posterior cortical atrophy and progressive supranuclear palsy.

The types of dementia listed earlier highlight a wealth of diverse experience and will be broadened given many other contributory factors such as the stage of the condition, personality characteristics, support mechanisms or the person's environment. When considering how many different types of dementia are there, it is perhaps worth acknowledging Kitwood's (1997) assertion of there being as many types of dementia as there are people with dementia. As the available narratives show, there are a multitude of varying experiences, uniquely different for each person. The experience is also subject to wide changes dependent upon the point in a person's journey with dementia.

FIRST SIGNS AND BEING TESTED

The first signs that something is wrong can be terrifying, bewildering and unsettling. Narrative accounts commonly illustrate a sense of growing concern, feelings of lurking terror and the experience of gradually losing one's grounding:

> For the first time in my life, doubt stirred somewhere deep inside. It was unsettling and unnerving, and for a time, I felt the uncertainty of a person experiencing a hurricane or a tornado for the first time: the terrifying sensation that comes on realizing that what should be firm and solid is no longer so, and cannot be relied upon.
>
> Rose (1996, p. 4)

This was coupled with the statement:

> Slowly and painfully, I was becoming aware of the darkness in my mind ... everything that is important to me in life is slowly slipping away.
>
> Rose (1996, p. 12)

Similarly, Barry Pankhurst (2014) highlights the emergent feelings of dread and helplessness:

> I remember reading that a person who was drowning said that life flashes before your eyes, well that's the feeling I have every day and every night with Alzheimer's. You continuously feel you are sinking into a quagmire that you can't get out of no matter how hard you fight, and as hard as your family and friends try to pull you out ... you only sink deeper in.

Narratives such as these illustrate the personal sense of terror connected with what is felt internally. There is a sense here that something is wrong although not knowing what. These experiences are symptomatic of many people's encounters although alarmingly, for a sizeable proportion of people, occur some years before help is finally sought (Chrisp et al., 2011). A study by Keady and Nolan (1995) demonstrated that the journey towards proper recognition of difficulties was a slow and cumbersome process with many rationalisations and excuses being applied. There are a number of reasons, for example, other than dementia which could cause a person to become more forgetful. This includes tiredness, stress, overwork, anxiety, depression, physical illnesses or the side effects of certain medications (Alzheimer's Society, 2013a). These aspects feature prominently in the

Alzheimer's Society's Talking Point forum with rationalisations and reassurances sought from other members:

> I'm scaring myself. It will be stress, yes?
>
> Alzheimer's Society (2011)

Graham (2012) describes how she in collusion with her husband avoided addressing their concerns:

> So for a while I came up with one crackpot explanation after another. I had a partner in this exercise of self-deception. One of the many lessons I've learned is that sufferers become very canny at patching over the holes. Questions that call for a precise answer get fudged.

The ability to make excuses or bluff one's way out of situations are evidently ways of coping with emergent fears and of trying to maintain a sense of 'normality'. A 2012 survey found that a third of people with dementia had waited longer than a year to go to their GP with their symptoms (All Party Parliamentary Group on Dementia, 2012). The reasons for this are complex and may include the assumption that memory problems are normal in older age, a fear of the diagnosis, a view that little can be done to help or the perceived stigma of dementia. The point of seeking help is in a number of cases initiated by the experience of a *decisive moment*, where the severity of symptoms cannot be overlooked (Nichols and Martindale-Adams, 2006). Such critical events provide individuals with a dramatic 'wake-up call' forcing them to address the extent of the problem (Hutchinson et al., 1997). The difficulty though in addressing what is going on is aptly summed up by Graham (2012):

> The terror dementia sufferers must feel is unimaginable but the techniques they use to hide their difficulties … are perfectly understandable … And you have dementia in a nutshell. The physician hesitates to name it, the sufferer denies he has it, and the carer's hair turns grey … Give Dementia time and she'll announce herself clearly enough.

BEING TESTED AND RECEIVING A DIAGNOSIS

> How would you feel if given a diagnosis of dementia?
>
> What implications would this have on your daily life?

Before receiving a dementia diagnosis, individuals have to first endure an arduous testing process which includes the MMSE (mental ability test), having blood taken, being put through a full physical examination and undergoing brain scans – computerised tomography (CT) and magnetic resonance imaging (NHS Choices, 2015). It is not hard to imagine that this will feel scary and exhausting as well as maybe bewildering and demeaning, something illustrated by Larry Rose (1996) who recounts how awkward and humiliated he felt at being unable to answer questions he reflected his 5-year-old grandson could easily manage. Diagnoses are being given now at much earlier stages and indeed the National Dementia Strategy (DoH, 2009) advocate practices which encourage early diagnosis and support. In the Facing Dementia Survey, a key finding showed that Alzheimer's disease remains undiagnosed until symptoms become moderate to severe because of the difficulties of recognising the early symptoms and the attributions of symptoms associated with normal ageing (Bond et al., 2005). The journey of Australian people with dementia and their carers was explored in the work of Speechly et al. (2008) who described a timeline of changes and events such as stopping driving, needing help with daily activities and contact with healthcare professionals. Their key findings were that it took almost 2 years to contact a healthcare professional and approximately 2.7 years from noticing symptom onset to receiving a diagnosis. Chrisp et al. (2011, p. 565) reported on the delays and decisions relating to early diagnosis:

> For those who reach the point of diagnosis, the mean journey time from thinking that something may be amiss to beginning the formal process of diagnosis is around three years.

Evidently, at the point of seeking professional help, undergoing the various tests available and then receiving a diagnosis individuals are no doubt already feeling drained, with many doubts and fears about their future. Trying to then conceptualise what the term *dementia* means or encapsulates will be a very arduous process with many fluctuating and conflicting emotions. The Alzheimer's Society provides a range of factsheets and booklets to support individuals on receiving a diagnosis such as their 'What your diagnosis means for you' booklet (Alzheimer's Society, 2010). This particular resource acknowledges feelings such as shock, disbelief, denial, fear, guilt and the sense of loss. There is no standard response to the receipt of a dementia diagnosis with each person having their own personal feelings about what it means to them. Richard Taylor (2007, p. 6), for example, viewed his Alzheimer's diagnoses as a devastating blow, referring to it as a 'spiral stairway to depression'. Similarly, Christine Bryden (2005), who was diagnosed with dementia in her late forties recounted the shock at receiving her diagnosis which felt like being cursed. This was heightened through the way it was given with the standard *dementia script* indicating the expected number of years she had left before having to enter a nursing home. She relates the great struggle in pretending that she was OK even though feeling as if she was

> Hanging onto a high cliff, above a lurking black hole.
>
> Bryden (2005, p. 98)

This initial sense of pessimism and hopelessness is reflected by Terry Pratchett's (2008) emotions and thoughts after receiving his dementia diagnosis:

> I remember on that day of rage thinking that if I'd been diagnosed with cancer of any kind, at least there would have opened in front of me a trodden path. There would have been specialists, examinations, there would be in short,

some machinery in place. I was not in the mood for a response that said, more or less, 'go away and come back in six years'. How brave is it to say you have a disease that does not hint of a dissolute youth, riotous living or even terrible eating habits?

This shows the very real care and sensitivity needed at the point of diagnosis and not fostering what Kate Swaffer (2012) refers to as prescribed disengagement:

Following diagnosis, my specialists all told me 'to give up work, give up study, and go home for the time I had left'!

People evidently need more information about what the term dementia actually means and examples of people living well with this condition. It is worth noting though that diagnosis be relieving for some people through obtaining a reason to account for the changes and difficulties they have been experiencing. An individual diagnosed with fronto-temporal dementia recounts finally having an answer for why the cutlery was in the washing machine and the phone under the grill (Alzheimer's Society, 2014b). Whilst this attempt at humour is clearly a means of coping with what will have also been an enormous and devastating shock, there is a sense of comprehension and sense-making of what has been occurring. The receipt of a diagnosis can have a significant personal impact with regards to thoughts about the future. A particularly poignant posting within the Alzheimer's Society's Talking Point Forum is the information shared by a person diagnosed with dementia in their 30s. This is particularly striking given the age of the individual concerned, having to face the reality of living with a condition normally associated with those who are much older. There is a sense of hopelessness and resignation being relayed in their narrative, signifying desperate needs for emotional and psychological support. It highlights the importance of having other people with whom one can talk to, share feelings and develop methods for coping with the changes and difficulties faced. Diana Friel McGowin (1993, p. 53) was diagnosed with Alzheimer's and multi infarct dementia at the age of 52. She relates feeling devastated and desperate for comfort and support from others:

What I wanted, no needed, was someone to assure me that no matter what my future held, they would stand by me, fight my battles with me, or of need be for me. I wanted assurance from someone that I would not be abandoned to shrivel away. They would give me encouragement, love, moral support, and if necessary, take care of me.

This vital expression illustrates the absolute terror of disappearing inside oneself, the feeling of helplessness and hopelessness about the future, the sense of becoming adrift and feeling isolated from others. It is not surprising therefore to note that lowered hope raises the potential for depression and suicide (Pinner, 2000; Tambini, 2008). The Dementia and Suicide Report, key point 10, states:

It may be the case that dementia is a risk factor for suicide in older people early in the course of the disease, when insight and the ability to plan and act are still present. Later in the course of the dementia the presence of the disease may be protective insofar as insight may be lost, the ability to plan suicide and act on the plan may be severely diminished, and there may be increased levels of supervision from carers and relatives.

Beeston (2006, p. 27)

Thoughts of taking one's own life strongly illustrate the magnitude of fear and hopelessness experienced by a number of people in the wake of a dementia diagnosis and the crucial need for effective support. As Woods et al. (2003) illustrate, this heightens concerns amongst practitioners who are fearful about the impact that a dementia diagnosis might have upon a person's flagging competence and fragile defences. As a consequence, diagnostic information is sometimes presented to individuals through general euphemisms such as 'memory difficulties' or other vague and poorly defined terms (Bamford et al., 2004; Downs et al., 2002). It is also the case that a number of people are not told at all, with relatives instead being informed. There are estimates of only half of people with dementia ever receiving a formal diagnosis (DoH, 2012). The holding back of information, whilst done paternalistically can be criticised because of the person's fundamental 'right to know' as well as not allowing them the opportunity to engage in future planning (Pinner, 2000). However, in Vernooij-Dassen et al.'s (2006) study, a number of participants felt that they would have preferred not to know due to the fears associated with the diagnosis. This raises a difficult and contentious area relating to how we might really know whether individuals wish to be informed or not and how we should respond.

YOUNG ONSET

The number of people in the United Kingdom with young-onset dementia is estimated to be over 40,000 (Alzheimer's Society, 2014a). Whilst dementia symptoms are similar across different age groups, the person's experience will be markedly different due to factors such as being in work at the time of diagnosis, having dependent children still living at home, having significant financial commitments and struggling to accept and cope with losing skills at such a young age (Alzheimer's Society, 2013c). Being diagnosed with dementia whilst still feeling young and productive can obviously be a huge shock, especially with a condition commonly regarded as 'an old person's disease'. It should be noted here though that feeling *old* is relative to the person with a number of people of advanced ages still being productive, fit and very able. There will be a similar impact made upon older people who have to contemplate similar restrictions to their activities and roles. The thoughts and feelings however for those diagnosed with young-onset dementia will include total bewilderment and shock in trying to contemplate what it means to their life. Clemerson et al. (2013) identified four themes impacting upon those with young-onset dementia:

- *Disruption of the life cycle*: This is related to a loss of adult competency and difficulties in fulfilling roles such as contributing to social groups or caring for the family.
- *Identity*: The onset of memory difficulties posed a threat to individuals' self-identity requiring a redefining of self in order to cope with future decline.

- *Social orientation*: There was a strong sense related of disconnection and isolation, enforced either by others or through the individual disengaging from social activities.
- *Agency*: Feelings of powerlessness and loss of agency were recounted with many participants sensing that they were no longer in control of their minds, actions, future and overall experiences.

The Alzheimer's Society's Talking Point forum features many postings from individuals with early onset dementia, concerned and seeking support. These postings illustrate something of the desperation and trepidation felt and the sheer sense of relief at finding people to share their feelings with. It is evident that significant emotional and psychological support will be needed, not just for the person diagnosed but also for their whole family.

'COMING OUT'

What would be your concerns about revealing a dementia diagnosis to others?

Who would you feel most able to talk to?

Who would you find it hardest to tell and why?

A significant and potentially very distressing moment for people with dementia concerns the point in time where others are informed of one's diagnosis. As Kate Swaffer (2013) noted reactions from others can vary between over-protectiveness, hostility (accusing you of lying) and denial. A sense of disbelief or dismissive reaction from others can be fairly common in the early stages when symptoms are less noticeable. Rationalisations or justifications can be offered such as 'I forget things too'. It can also be the case if a person is of a younger age that others struggle to acknowledge the presence of what they see as an older person's condition. Taylor (2007), for example, found many people simply not believing that he had been diagnosed with dementia because he was not behaving in the way somebody with Alzheimer's was expected to. Similarly, Christine Bryden (2005) found herself when speaking at conferences having to show pictures of her own brain scan as a means of convincing others of the legitimacy of her diagnosis. Whilst talking to others about one's diagnosis can feel liberating and lead to much needed support, people can also experience difficulties relating to the lowered expectations commonly held regarding dementia. As a consequence individuals might be selective in who to tell or guarded in how much to reveal. Taylor (2007) felt the need to disguise his condition with initially only close friends and family members being aware. He continued to work as a teacher for a few years before withdrawing from his employment. This highlights a core difficulty where 'coming out' has different perceived consequences of role dependent upon who is being told, with employers being a particularly difficult group to broach. Fears about telling others include the worry of being seen as different to the person one was pre-diagnosis as well as subsequently being defined predominantly through one's diagnosis.

LOSS

One of the biggest problem areas facing those with dementia relates to the difficulty in having to deal with loss. Losses can be multifaceted and include aspects such as work and leisure pursuits, independence, status, function, memory role, ability, social sphere, and most poignantly self. These have profound implications upon a person's emotional and psychological well-being. They can also become a predominant perceptual feature whereby other people focus more upon what those with dementia *can't do* as opposed to what they *can do* (Sabat, 2001). This conceptualises dementia as a defining entity, something which overshadows a person and causes them to be viewed from a perspective of increasing helplessness, risk and incapability. As well as shaping the attitudes held by others, there is likely to be a degree of internalisation of critical and doubtful thoughts by those with dementia. If, for example, we are regularly questioned about what we are able to do we will gradually come to feel less secure about our own abilities.

Social contact and work are spheres in which losses are keenly felt. Isolation is a significant problem with a person's social life gradually becoming eroded. It contributes to the perception of a 'shrinking world' and developing detachment from others. Responses from others, difficulties in communicating, anxieties and fears as well as lowered self-esteem can all play a part in a person's progressive withdrawal or alienation. Lowered expectations and stereotypical associations will also negatively influence things. Brittain et al. (2010) found that familiar environments enabled individuals to carry on with everyday activities whilst outside space was perceived as frightening with individuals feeling 'out of place'. This clearly contributes towards the decreasing range of involvement a person has with others. An initiative aimed at promoting social contact and inclusion in daily life is the Alzheimer's Society's Dementia Friends initiative. There are many positive elements to this with inclusion of a driving factor and the need for agencies and organisations to be aware of potential problems in daily life. Ken Clasper (2014) applauds initiatives such as a bus company's colour coding of buses and painting routes on the side. However,

> there are days when these same buses are used in totally different areas and routes ... the operators simply do not understand the confusion they are causing.

Similar issues have no doubt been witnessed in numerous care facilities with orientation aids displaying dates, seasons and other information not kept updated, in some instances significantly so.

Loss can also relate to work, something which occupies a large part of people's lives, providing status, security, social contact and feelings of productivity. Having to give up work through infirmity can make a person feel useless as expressed by Friel-McGowin (1993), who struggled for a while to prolong her working life with various temping jobs before reluctantly and upsettingly finally having to stop. Another significant loss of ability making a person feel useless and helpless concerns the need to give up driving. This can impact strongly upon a person's sense of independence as related strongly by individuals in the Alzheimer's Society's Talking Point Forum, relating feelings of anger, humiliation and helplessness. This illustrates the sense of enforced dependency and increasing restrictiveness a person feels when having to stop doing things and rely more upon others. We can imagine then the sense of anxious anticipation as to what is next to be lost or taken away, even with everyday activities. This is powerfully highlighted by Davis (1989, p. 103):

> I live with the imminent dread that one mistake in my daily life will mean another freedom will be taken from me … For example, any housewife can forget a pan on the stove and burn dinner. She and her family just laugh about it and get a can of something else out for supper … for the person with Alzheimer's it may be the end to a whole line of productivity.

A common response from others is to offer help and support to limit the difficulties experienced. Whilst some people might assume that support if needed will be welcomed, it can feel an intrusion or threat to a person's remaining faculties and abilities. This is powerfully expressed by Bryden (2005, p. 103):

> If you take over our lives then it is easy for us to withdraw into helplessness. Life is so hard anyway and you can make it much easier for us … but in so doing we will lose functions.

Our interests, likes and dislikes, the experiences we have had, the jobs we do, our circle of family and friends and the roles we adopt all play a significant part in defining who we are. Losses in these areas will slowly erode one's identity and feel devastating. Perhaps the most terrifying and devastating loss concerns the loss of what makes us who we are, or more specifically loss of self. The perception of respondents in Goldsmith's (1996) study was that dementia was destroying the personalities of their loved ones. The notion that the *person within* is no longer there causes great despair to individuals with dementia as well as family and friends (Kitwood, 1997). For the person with dementia, there are many fears and uncertainties about the future, as eloquently expressed by Voyager in the Alzheimer's Society's (2005, p. 2) *Living with Dementia* magazine:

> Like Columbus, I am on a voyage of discovery. My route is not exact and I must make adjustments as I go along … unlike being at sea in a storm, I know that the voyage is only going to become more difficult. It may become a typhoon or hurricane, depending on where it takes me. This storm will not pass: I have to make suitable preparations before the force 12 hits. Let me tell you that I am lucky: I have very good friends who will be with me on the stormy ride ahead.

Voyager's narrative expressively highlights the anticipated journey into unexplored territory, travelling without maps or any navigable aids. There is a sense here of exchanging the known for the unknown, which will be scary and unsettling. The sentiments being expressed here are reflected in Harman and Clare's (2006) study which investigated illness representations in early-stage dementia, finding two overarching themes of *it will get worse* and *I want to be me*. This encapsulates the terror one must feel when losing precious memories such as the birth of one's children or one's wedding day. There is also the tragedy in contemplating a time when one's family and friends, lifetime experiences, moments of triumph and joy or perhaps favourite songs gradually recede away and become lost. There can be an absolute need here for others to retain a sense of *what it means to be me*. This reflects a commonly expressed request for trusted advocates to safeguard and retain a person's memories for them, to represent and promote what is *vital* about them on their behalf.

> Think of your three most precious memories.
>
> Next, consider giving one of them away.
>
> How does this make you feel?

ENGAGEMENT ISSUES

Another important and striking difficulty relates to communicative deficits and impaired engagement with others. Problems here fuel feelings of disconnectedness and the perception of occupying a 'shrinking world'. The ability to communicate provides individuals with a voice, a means of connecting and engaging with others and the ability to feel accepted and understood. It is something which is commonly affected in dementia with words progressively losing their meaning or significance. This is illustrated by Silverfox (2014b) who recounts struggling to locate the right word with his mouth, lips and tongue refusing to work together. Communication is also experienced as problematic with letters appearing jumbled or absent from words making comprehension difficult. A posting in the Alzheimer's Society Talking Point Forum states:

> I now have speech problems ... when I go to reply the mind and voice becomes frozen and all that comes out is a slurred stammering, yes the words of a reply are within me but they won't come out which then makes me even more frustrated and bewildered and I often end up in tears, yes a grown man in tears.

> Alzheimer's Society (2015a)

This reflects a very distressing experience, with words and meaning locked inside infuriatingly out of reach by others. The impairment in communication (both conveying and receiving messages) will have a striking impact upon a person leading to the diminishment of their engagement with things external to them and their sphere of influence. As a consequence of this an individual is prone to becoming more detached and withdrawn. The culmination of this process is the perceived state of 'vegetation', illustrated by Naomi Feil (2012) as a point of total disengagement from the world around them. The process of engagement with others just becomes too difficult. This is evidently a desperately lonely place to impacting upon opportunities for intimacy, one of the most important aspects for a person with dementia. Intimacy relates to a central need for closeness and attachment, aspects which are strongly impacted upon through dementia with individuals feeling progressively more isolated and disconnected (Kitwood, 1997). Alongside the emotional and psychological dimensions, there is a physical need as illustrated by Kate Swaffer (2015a):

> Just because we have dementia does not mean we don't want to have sex.

She also highlights the notable absence of people with dementia as speakers at a forthcoming conference on sex and dementia. This is significant and highlights an aspect with which professional carers are clearly uncomfortable. Within clinical settings opportunities for intimate contact between partners or indeed non-partners can be low. Concerns around competence, vulnerability and risk can be lead practitioners to be overly cautious or even dismissive of service users' needs.

PHYSICAL CHANGES AND DAILY FUNCTIONING

It is important initially that physical problems contributing to confusional states are ruled out such as infection, constipation, hormonal imbalance or inadequate nutrition (Kitwood, 1997). The fact that a large number of those with dementia are of advanced age means that a significant number are living with declining physical abilities which affect mobility, vision and hearing. They may also have to contend with the co-existence of other conditions such as strokes impacting upon functioning such as communication, eating and drinking or mobility. Mobility problems are commonly experienced in dementia affecting balance and coordination with a range of movements gradually becoming more impacted upon. Valerie Blumenthal (2014) describes her fear of descending steps and stairs:

> As they swayed before me I morphed into a scared old woman, clinging on to the railings for dear life. The stairs existed solely for me to break my neck. And as for escalators, I confronted these with horror. I could not get the timing right and lurched onto them, getting my feet sandwiched between the treads.

Experiences such as this are liable to make a person feel awkward, embarrassed, foolish and terrified. It is likely to result in restricting and limiting a person's desire to go out and engage in activities. Rose (1996) reflected upon his experience of having to cling to the backs of chairs to maintain his balance, whilst distressingly overhearing someone relate to him as a 'drunk'. Symptoms of dementia such as confusion, slurred speech, unsteady gait and difficulties with self-care can all mimic signs of alcohol intoxication. Receiving critical or disparaging comments from others about being intoxicated will be hurtful and will negatively impact upon a person's flagging confidence levels.

Another significant physical manifestation caused by the extended effort needed to function with dementia is that of exhaustion. The extra levels of concentration and attention needed even for everyday tasks such as walking or simply holding a drink without spilling are regarded by Bryden (2005) as being physically draining. Greater time is needed to complete tasks and process information as is space for rest and recuperation. Davis (1989) remembers a family holiday to Disney World which left him feeling overwhelmed and with a crucial need to retreat to a quiet space, in this instance to a darkened room, where he remained for days before being able to regain his ability to function. The world for him had simply become too demanding and strenuous to cope with. Whilst he had the ability and freedom to satisfy his need for space and solitude there are very real implications concerning those who do not have the ability to communicate or act upon their needs.

DEPRESSION

Studies have found over 70% of those with dementia experiencing depressive symptoms at some stage during their illness (Starkstein, 2014; Tractenberg et al., 2003). It is not surprising that the difficulties associated with dementia impact upon a person's mood given the multiple losses experienced and profound changes in status, role and functioning. As Kitwood (1997) states, depression is common in the aftermath of a dementia diagnosis owing to its fearful connotations. This is reflected by the heightened risk of suicide in those newly diagnosed with dementia (Seyfried et al., 2011). Mental health states such as depression and anxiety mask some of the symptoms of dementia making accurate assessment difficult. This is highlighted by Insel and Badger (2002) concerning a person's depressed mood making their state of cognitive decline appear more pronounced. Symptoms common to both depression and dementia include apathy, loss of interest in activities and hobbies, social withdrawal, isolation, trouble concentrating and impaired thinking (Alzheimer's Society, 2014c). A clear example of the association between depression and cognitive difficulties is provided by Christine Bryden (2005, p. 17):

> I had really deteriorated, changing as a person, losing the super-fast, super-smart me. I had become much slower in my speech, less able to make decisions, and more readily confused … I was well into my journey with the disease, experiencing most of the cognitive, behavioural and neurological signs of mild to moderate dementia. I no longer drove, answered the phone or watched TV, but retreated into gardening and books, as well as early bedtimes.

This narrative might appear normal with regard to expectations around dementia; however, there were changes as her mood lifted (p. 18):

> My head began to clear of the fuzzy 'cotton wool' type of feeling that it felt like before. I could concentrate better, and found it easier to speak and listen.

She reflects upon her symptoms here as a form of pseudo-dementia, which as outlined by Gainotti and Marra (1994) can mimic a depressive episode. Where a person has depression (loss of interest and pleasure in daily activities, social withdrawal, sleep and appetite disturbances) and cognitive symptoms (difficulties in thinking clearly, problems concentrating and difficulties in making decisions), they may appear to exhibit signs and symptoms of dementia. This highlights the importance of looking beyond observed symptoms and challenging assumptions and expectations around the condition of dementia. The impact that depression has upon a person such as decreased mood, apathy, poor concentration and withdrawal might all be easily mistaken as symptoms and signs of cognitive deterioration. It is important therefore to correctly identify and treat underlying depression as attributing deterioration in functioning solely to a person's dementia can result in lowered expectations and a further reinforcement of despondency and helplessness. Whilst depression is commonly experienced by individuals with dementia it is important to note that this is not the case for everyone, nor is it a constant state for those who are affected. As will be seen later, many people continue to live well or experience feelings of well-being despite the presence of dementia in their lives.

ANXIETY

In what ways could having dementia affect your confidence and make you more fearful?

How might this impact upon your daily life?

The steady decline in cognitive ability has the impact of causing individuals to feel less sure of themselves and the world in which they live. This experience can be linked with increased states of confusion and difficulties in processing information. Phinney (2002) highlighted the fear and uncertainty felt by individuals on finding themselves in unfamiliar places and situations. This is liable to cause people to withdraw from activities and isolate themselves from others, retreating to a place of 'safety' or what feels familiar. The feelings of uncertainty and disquiet can be hard to escape from in what can feel like a steadily fragmenting world. Indeed, Taylor (2007) described his worries using a volcano as a metaphor with fear represented by the magma deep inside waiting to erupt. Anxiety disorders are commonly associated with dementia, particularly where insight is retained (Ballard et al., 1994). As with depression, it can be difficult to distinguish between anxiety and dementia symptoms with an overlap of features commonly noted (Shankar and Orrell, 2000). A person's stress tolerance is lowered with dementia and as Bryden (2005) recounts even minor disruptions can cause a catastrophic reaction with the need to shout, scream, panic or pace about. Dealing with pent-up feelings and agitation can be related to wandering behaviour, something which Davis (1989, p. 109) reflects upon:

When the darkness and emptiness fill my mind, it is totally terrifying … thoughts increasingly haunt me. The only way to break this cycle is to move.

He indicates the necessity for engaging in productive, physically demanding activities, something clearly restricted for many people in residential care facilities. Anxiety states can reflect something of a person's inner feelings, reframing a number of observed 'challenging behaviours' such as agitation, attention seeking and wandering. Anxiety states are often perceived as agitation, a very common expression experienced by around 60% of people with dementia at some stage through their illness (Mintzer and Brawman-Mintzer, 1996). The impact of anxiety upon a person's functioning can be profound. This can relate to decreased social engagement, lowered confidence, withdrawal from activities and enhanced dependency.

The lowered expectations that are generally applied to people with dementia are heavily reinforced and are likely to become internalised with thoughts of 'maybe I can't do this'. A person's declining cognitive functioning will make everyday activities and social interactions more arduous and anxiety provoking influencing a person's withdrawal. There is a need therefore for carers to show sensitivity towards underlying anxiety states or feelings of uncertainty and offer a range of supportive interventions, wider than merely using pharmaceutical agents.

SECTION 2: EXPERIENCING SUPPORT

Interview narratives

Where I live, sheltered housing, there are staff who work there and they come and wake me up in the morning. They always bring me a cup of coffee and a bowl of cornflakes. I'm happy with that.

There's other people here [Day Centre] and everybody knows what you're going through. It's a big help and they're fabulous the people here... not alone is important.

What I feel is needed more than anything else is patience ... I've got this problem up at the home with one of the staff ... she talks to you like an idiot, not like a person but an idiot who doesn't know anything.

Here it's so they different, they all understand. I just love coming here because the staff are fantastic and you can talk to them about any worries you've got.

Whilst a selection of narratives exist detailing subjective experience of various supportive interventions, some approaches such as residential care are harder to evidence owing to a person's deteriorating communicative ability. There will however be a reflection upon how support is experienced with regard to psychological therapies, medication, in-patient/residential care, creative arts, reminiscence, validation and peer support.

PSYCHOLOGICAL THERAPIES

What psychological support do you feel is needed for people living with dementia?

When should this type of support be offered and to whom?

It is important for psychotherapeutic approaches to address the totality of a person's experience with dementia. This looks beyond the physical changes taking place in the brain and acknowledges the psychological and emotional manifestations present. The urgent need for emotional support is indicated through many narratives as reflected by Silverfox (2015a):

When someone asks me how I am doing, I normally say I am as well as I can be. That of course is a lie!

This blog continues expressing feelings of being lost and isolated, disconnected, grumpy, agitated and angry, desperately needing someone to talk with. Bryden (2002) regards the behaviours seen in dementia as adaptive responses to the experience of cognitive decline, rather than directly the result of brain pathology. She argues therefore that a variety of psychotherapeutic interventions such as grief counselling, non-directive counselling, long-term supportive psychodynamic psychotherapy, cognitive-behavioural therapy and rehabilitation are required. This would address a range of psychological and emotional problems such as depression, anger, anxiety, hopelessness and grief. Counselling and psychotherapy can also be useful in helping individuals with dementia make sense of how their lives are changing, understand more about how they are feeling, identify available support mechanisms and learn how to cope with their condition more effectively (Alzheimer's Society, 2015b). Hill and Brettle (2005) report on a review carried out by the British Association for Counselling and Psychotherapy finding counselling to be efficacious in the treatment of anxiety and depression amongst individuals with dementia. Bender and Cheston's (1997) study investigated the subjective world of people with dementia sufferers and found experiences of anxiety, depression, grief, despair and terror all supporting the need for using psychotherapy. Various forms of psychotherapy have been offered to individuals with dementia as well as less-verbal intervention such as music and art therapy (Bonder, 1994). The range of approaches available can be helpful at different stages in a person's dementia journey. This is particularly the case for people newly diagnosed with dementia and requiring support in working through denial of the diagnosis and feelings of grief connected with the experience of actual or anticipated losses (Aminzadeh et al., 2007). Psychotherapeutic interventions can be effective in helping people with dementia adjust to the effects of their illness (Junaid and Hegde, 2007), reduce levels of depression (Cheston and Jones, 2009) and relieve some of the behavioural and psychological symptoms of dementia (Ericson and Eriksson, 2013). Watkins et al. (2006) report on a project investigating changes that occurred for participants during a series of time-limited psychotherapy groups for people with dementia. One participant, reflecting on the changes that had occurred for him commented that before he came to the group he had been frightened, worrying that

I'm going crazy ... what am I going to be like in another five years?

Through attendance of the group, his fear was consoled with the acknowledgement that he was not alone and he was assisted in dealing with his feelings of being 'different'. This shows one of the important elements of group therapy, feeling connected and understood by others who are sharing similar experiences (Yalom, 2005). It can be noted that whilst groups can be useful in reducing levels of depression and anxiety, they are most effective within mild to moderate dementia and are not suitable for all people with dementia (Cheston et al., 2003).

MEDICATION

There are a number of pharmaceutical treatments used within dementia care. Acetylcholinesterase inhibitors (Aricept, Exelon and Reminyl) maintain existing supplies of acetylcholine in the brain, whilst another medication, Ebixa, blocks a messenger chemical known as glutamate which causes damage to brain cells. These medication types are recommended for people in both moderate and severe stages of Alzheimer's disease (Alzheimer's Society, 2014d). These treatments according to NICE (2011) should be continued only when it is considered to be having a worthwhile effect on cognitive, global, functional or behavioural symptoms. This is challenged by a number of postings on the Alzheimer's Society's Talking Point Forum with people unhappy about this approach and feeling that there also exists a form of postcode lottery. The NICE (2011) guidance recommends that for mild to moderate Alzheimer's disease (MMSE score 10–26) a person should be considered for treatment with one of the acetylcholinesterase inhibitors with memantine (Ebixa) offered to some of those with moderate disease (MMSE score 10–20) or severe Alzheimer's disease (MMSE score less than 10).

> How would you feel if informed by your Dr that your medication would not be pre-scribed anymore as it would not offer you any further discernible benefits?

Discussion threads on the Alz Connected discussion forum from people taking medication for dementia highlight day-to-day problems with side effects. A particular issue is experienced by those taking Aricept and problems with nausea and diarrhoea. Other side effects from taking medication for dementia are reflected by bloggers. Glick (2014) noted feeling tired and apathetic with a rise in his energy levels after discontinuing his medication (memantine). Silverfox (2015b) recounted:

> [over] the last few days, I have really been disconnected and cognitively slow. This may be from my change to Namenda XR, or it may be a new progression of the disease. I just do not know.

This was weighed up against worries around not taking medication and deteriorating faster. An issue being reflected here though concerns the added uncertainty around what the possible contributory factors impacting upon one's symptoms might be.

Worries about appropriate medication prescribing are particularly connected with the over-prescribing of sedative or antipsychotic medication within dementia care (Barnes et al., 2012). Whilst there may be short-term benefits from using such medication to treat psychological and behavioural symptoms, there are some serious potential risks including strokes and increased mortality (Ballard and Howard, 2006). It was also found that giving neuroleptic medication to agitated individuals with Alzheimer's made their condition worse and was associated with a marked deterioration in verbal skills after just 6 months of treatment (Ballard et al., 2008). For the person with dementia, psychological and behavioural symptoms such as agitation are a means of communicating distress and need understanding with internal feelings or 'drivers' being responded to. In many cases, medication will not address internal feelings but instead reduce an individual's ability to express their distress.

IN-PATIENT AND RESIDENTIAL CARE

Understanding lived experience when receiving residential care is particularly difficult to fathom due to deteriorating communicative abilities. It can in part be appreciated through Kitwood and Bredin's (1992) *marks of well-being* and the associated *Dementia Care Mapping* which evaluate a person over a period of time concerning their engagement with their environment. The fact that individuals may be experiencing difficulties can be ascertained from the numerous reports and observations of a person's 'challenging behaviour' which is indicative of internal distress. An aspect to consider with regard to residential care concerns how people feel about being looked after. An assumption which may be applied to older people is that of *desired dependence*, the feeling that they would naturally welcome being looked after. Whilst this may be the case for some people, for others it can threaten dwindling capabilities and foster feelings of frustration and helplessness. A number of these aspects can be regarded as direct consequences of less-effective care practices included within Kitwood's (1997) *malignant social psychology* factors. Although often done in a paternalistic and caring way these care approaches fail to acknowledge the subjective experience or individuality of the person being worked with and have a seriously detrimental impact. Tom Kitwood (1997) identified a series of person-centred interventional approaches which he called *enhancing personhood* factors. This is illustrated in the work also being done by David Sheard, a specialist consultant in dementia care, which combines what may be regarded as plain common sense with creative approaches to help people with dementia retain a meaningful and active engagement with their environment (Dementia Care Matters, 2015).

A particular area of concern with regard to residential care concerns perceived areas of risk, where fears about a person's safety (or resultant litigation) result in various restrictions being implemented. Risk-taking is part of everyday life and needs to be addressed in a sensitive and reasoned way. This was illustrated very strongly in the TV documentary *Can Gerry Robinson Fix Dementia Care Homes* (Camden, 2009) where requests for residents to have their environment brightened and plants added were challenged with concerns such as the residents might eat the plants. The response by David Sheard to care home staff illustrated greater clarity of thinking considering the greater harm which might be caused to residents through boredom, lack of stimulation and inactivity. This strongly illustrates the point that greater education and training is needed for those working in dementia care to understand more about how people feel about and interact with their environment.

Other aspects to consider involve choice and opportunities for independent activity. People generally have their own personal range of coping mechanisms to respond to emotions such as sadness, irritability, loneliness or uncertainty. This might include seeking other people out, listening to a particular song, engaging in vigorous activity or finding a space of peace and solitude. If unable to satisfy these needs or communicate them to others a person is much more liable to exhibit what can be perceived as problem behaviours. Davis (1989) writes expressively about ways he copes with distressing internal feelings such as retreating to a quiet darkened room or engaging in strenuous exercise. Having the ability to satisfy these needs was regarded as essential to him in helping to retain a feeling of equilibrium. This raises real concerns for care home residents with impaired communicative ability who are unable to gain relief or support from others and are left with their distress.

It is interesting to note the thoughts from a number of people with dementia considering their own residential care at some point in the future. Phelps (2014) found having discussions with his wife about future placements helping to reduce anxieties about the future. Similarly, Chris Roberts (2014b) relates:

> Well after a long search, a very long search Iive finally found a care home, one with Wi-Fi I might add which is very difficult to find... At least now I got somewhere that I can go and have a day off once a week, time off from being me, time off from being on duty at home where the wife and children expect me to be me!... Just sat in a care home I can switch off completely, become no one! which I think will help to my stress levels, my idea is for every couple of days completely stress free will give me a few more days on the end total.

This is significant and illustrates a positive and supportive aspect connected with residential care facilities, reducing the levels of demand or expectation which a person can otherwise feel overwhelmed with. It reflects narratives previously covered showing how individuals can become fatigued and drained through continuous requirements to process information. Obviously the importance is in achieving the right balance for each individual and their families where respite and support can be obtained whilst promoting maximum functioning.

CREATIVE ARTS

Cogito ergo sum ('I think, therefore I am', or better translated as 'I am thinking, therefore I exist') is a philosophical proposition expressed by René Descartes (Open University, 2015). It means that thoughts about one's existence prove that an 'I' exists to do the thinking. Common assumptions that the person with dementia has disappeared and that we are left with simply a physical entity relate to the difficulties in connecting with and reaching the individual inside. It is clear though that we need to question our attempts to reach and connect with the person who is experiencing dementia. Creative and expressive modes can be very beneficial here re-engaging and reawakening the person inside. This has been shown through innovative and creative approaches such as the Meet me at Museum of Modern Art (MoMA) project or the Alzheimer's Society's Singing for the Brain initiative which bring people with dementia and their partners together with powerful results noted. Many positive responses have been received, for example, from those taking part in the Singing for the Brain groups with statements denoting pleasure, satisfaction and feeling being better connected and engaged with others. Positive feelings were also indicated by those with advanced dementia through non-verbal means such as smiling, greater movement and sense of vitality, aspects which were regarded as being at odds with how they were described at other times (NHS Choices, 2014).

The response from using arts-based activities can sometimes seem miraculous with individuals with advanced dementia seemingly becoming *reanimated* and regaining contact with their external environment. This was observed by Basting (2006) with people who had previously withdrawn into themselves and shut themselves off from the world around them. The arts enabled them to reconnect not only with themselves but also with people within their external environment. The range of arts-based activities used within dementia care is extensive with positive results found, for example, with poetry (Aadlandsvik, 2008), art (Zeisl, 2009), music (Aldridge, 1994) and dance (Duignan et al., 2009). The *Creative Dementia Arts Network* reports upon a number of projects including the Creative Minds programme which incorporates more than 180 creative projects. These have particularly worked well, with people who have traditionally been difficult to engage. There are many such initiatives being used nationally and worldwide to positive effect. The beneficial use of art with people with dementia was shown in Rusted et al.'s (2006) multicentre randomised control group trial on the use of art therapy for people with dementia. This provided clear evidence of changes in mental alertness, sociability, physical and social engagement.

REMINISCENCE

Mills' (1997) study found memories to be strongly linked with narrative identity and stressed the importance of reminiscence work in terms of retaining a sense of self. The process of reminiscence is essentially about recalling past experiences and 'bringing memories to life' (Age Exchange). Structured reminiscence can be beneficial in terms of stimulating a person's interest and enjoyment as well as helping to reinforce their identity and self-esteem (Schweitzer and Bruce, 2008; Wang, 2007). There have been some creative and valuable reminiscence projects geared towards stimulating shared recollections of life within people's localities. An example of this relates to an innovative reminiscence project concerning football recollections and experiences. Participants in Schofield and Tolson's (2010) study related a number of benefits from being part of this group as well as their enjoyment at attending with the company and camaraderie especially valued. It was noted that some participants spoke in groups, with partners relating that they had previously been silent and unresponsive for weeks or months. Various resources such as photographs of players and matches triggered animated discussion. There was a feeling that these reminiscence groups helped remind individuals about things which had meaning for them and contributed towards an increase in confidence and well-being. What is important here concerns the reaching out to people and re-engaging them through memories which resonate with them. This can be done in a number of ways with moments rekindled through photographs and film, music and songs, smells, tastes or textures. Each person will have their own set of sensations which if engaged with can provide a powerful connection to memories, experiences and feelings which have personal meaning for them.

VALIDATION

Validation therapy was developed by Naomi Feil (2012) for older people with cognitive impairments and is based upon accepting the reality and personal truth of another's experience. It can be regarded as a humane, practical approach based on knowledge about and empathy for the progressively isolating plight of the dementia sufferer, emphasising stage-specific communication techniques (Jones, 1977). Neal and Barton Wright (2009) reviewed the available research investigating the effectiveness of validation therapy. They concluded that there was insufficient evidence from randomised trials to draw any reliable conclusions about the efficacy of validation therapy. However, there have been many illustrations from practice which make this an approach worth considering. Perhaps one of the most potent can be observed on YouTube with a video showing Feil sharing a breakthrough moment in communication with Gladys Wilson, a woman diagnosed with Alzheimer's and particularly closed off from her external environment. It illustrates how Feil establishes a real sense of connection through singing, touch, proximity and matching her rhythm with that of Gladys.

ASSISTIVE TECHNOLOGY

Initiatives aimed at supporting independent living involve a range of technological resources known as assistive technology. These services provide devices which monitor activity, assess risks in a person's environment, predict problems and alert professional carers (Alzheimer's Society, 2015c). Other resources provide reminders and assist with orientation. One individual, involved in trialling various resources comments upon the beneficial functions of a memory prompt App which when pointed at people informs the user who they are (Which Me Am I Today, 2015). Comments are also made about the App's reminder facility and its usefulness for daily life. It is regarded as an exciting resource as well as one which is accessible and learnable.

The importance of services and functions such as these concerns the maintenance of independent living and the promotion of well-being. As further technological resources are created new benefits can be attained; however, these should be seen as complementary interventions and not simply as a substitute for approaches involving people.

PEER SUPPORT

How important do you feel it is to have contact with other people experiencing and living with dementia?

A major means of support, engagement and comfort is provided by peers – other people who have dementia. This involves individuals who are expertly placed to understand what a person with dementia might be experiencing. There are a number of community groups, online forums and support networks available including dementia cafes, self-help resources and internet discussion groups. A vital and highly valued resource is the Alzheimer's Society's Talking Point forum. This provides individuals with opportunities to share information, feel connected and heard as well as to support each other. Within the sections available, the *support from other members* area has thousands of discussion threads arranged under a variety of headings such as *recently diagnosed with dementia*. The number of people posting queries or replying to others shows widespread use with a high level of support evidenced, for example:

Wishing you a warm welcome to TP. I hope you'll find the forum as helpful as I have—it's been a Godsend often.

This is reflected in numerous other postings which indicate how important it feels to be able to share one's experiences and feelings with people who understand.

The responses given in this forum are helpful, empathic and supportive. The sharing of information and engagement with others is vital in combating the isolation and disconnection strongly felt in dementia. It is evident that connection with others who are seen to be in a similar position is an immense support and provides a vital sense of connectedness and hope.

SECTION 3: LIVING BEYOND DEMENTIA (SWAFFER, 2015C)

Interview narratives

I do a lot with the puzzle books and it's good for my head. Well it's like exercise, exercise for your brain isn't it, it stimulates it.

I think it's about letting your family know and your family can then help you which my daughter does.

At home in my kitchen I have one of those boards and I write on what I'm going to do and when I'm going to do and when I've done it I tick it off. And same again for next day.

I still do the things I did before.

Do you feel it is possible to live well with dementia?

A point to challenge is the common belief that those with dementia must be in distress and *suffering with dementia*. Whilst acknowledging some of the distressing and life changing aspects that people experience along with some very real despair it is important to note the successes, pleasurable experiences and new learning which can also be experienced. The sense of life continuing despite the presence of dementia is reflected within a number of narratives. Leah (2007), for example, determinedly asserts that despite being diagnosed with early-onset dementia, she still has a life to live. This statement highlights a resolve to fight on and maintain her quality of life. Terry Pratchett (2008) substitutes the term 'a person who is thoroughly annoyed with the fact they have dementia' for that of dementia sufferer. When looking at this moniker there is a presupposition that depressive feelings are constant, which is not the case. Further challenge to this is given by Kate Swaffer (2015b) who challenges the label *dementia sufferer* stating that she wants to be allowed to live with hope and attain the best life possible.

Feelings of well-being are subject to change and can be present at any stage within a person's dementia journey. An aspect to consider concerns that of ability. Harman and Clare (2006) reflect the coping stance taken by those experiencing dementia as lying on a continuum between self-maintaining responses (aimed at maintaining the prior sense of self and seeing problems as normal part of ageing) and self-adjusting responses (acknowledging the changes dementia brings and integrating them into one's sense of identity). This helps to shift the focus from a *deficits-led* perspective to what might be regarded as an *abilities-led* approach.

Postings on the Alzheimer's Society's Talking Point Forum convey very strongly the sense of the dementia experience being mixed with optimism and resilience expressed alongside feelings of helplessness and despair. Terry Pratchett (2008) expressed this dichotomy with feelings of distress:

> 'I'm slipping away a bit at a time ... and all I can do is watch it happen', combined with a sense of determination, 'The first step is to talk openly about dementia because it's a fact, well enshrined in folklore, that if we are to kill the demon then first we have to say its name'.

This reinforces the aspect that doubt, uncertainty and despair need not necessarily be representative of one's total journey, something expressed very eloquently by Christine Bryden (2005, p. 170), a noted dementia campaigner:

> I choose a new identity as a survivor. I want to learn to dance with dementia. I want to live positively each day, in a vital relationship of trust with my care partners alongside me.

She further added (p. 11):

> Each person with dementia is travelling a journey deep into the core of their spirit, away from the complex outer layer that once defined them, through the jumble and tangle of emotions created through their life experiences, into the centre of their being, into what truly gives them meaning in life.

This need to carry on despite advancing difficulties is supported by Ken Clasper (2014) who stresses the importance of taking each day as it comes and to try and enjoy life as much as possible. It is clear that this is a sentiment shared by many people with dementia as evidenced by the Alzheimer's Society's *Living with Dementia* magazine which documents numerous stories of success, productivity and ability post-diagnosis, such as running marathons, writing books, speaking at conferences and even getting married. The sense of determination to live one's life is reflected by Max McCormick (2015) who stresses that the difficulties he faces are only part of his total experience and that he will not be prevented from doing the things that he still can do. A final thought concerning this can be given to Kate Swaffer (2015c) who advocates the use of the term *living beyond dementia*. This importantly encapsulates positivity and continuity of life, which can include fresh challenges, new ventures and further achievements.

Dementia therefore need not define the totality of a person's life. The narratives reviewed in this chapter have been humbling, instructional and inspiring and provide much food for thought when considering the lived experience of those living with dementia.

REFERENCES

Aadlandsvik, R. (2008). The second sight. Learning about and with dementia by means of poetry. *Dementia*. 7(3), 321–329.

Age Exchange. (2015). Reminiscence. http://www.age-exchange.org.uk/, accessed 22 September, 2015.

Aldridge, D. (1994). Alzheimer's disease: Rhythm, timing and music as therapy. *Biomedicine & Pharmacotherapy*. 48(7), 275–281.

All Party Parliamentary Group on Dementia (2012). *Unlocking Diagnosis: The Key to Improving the Lives of People with Dementia*. Alzheimer's Society: London, UK.

Alzheimer's Society. (2015). Talking Point forum. http://forum.alzheimers.org.uk/, accessed 16 June, 2015.

Alzheimer's Society (2005). Navigating the sea of dementia. http://forum.alzheimers. org.uk, accessed 22 September, 2015.

Alzheimer's Society (2008). Talking Point forum. http://forum.alzheimers.org.uk/, accessed 3 June, 2015.

Alzheimer's Society (2010). *What Your Diagnosis Means to You*. Alzheimer's Society: London, UK.

Alzheimer's Society (2011). Talking Point forum. http://forum.alzheimers.org.uk/, accessed 16 June, 2015.

Alzheimer's Society (2013a). About dementia. http://www.alzheimers.org.uk/, accessed 16 June, 2015.

Alzheimer's Society (2013b). 37 diagnosed. http://forum.alzheimers.org.uk/, accessed 18 June, 2015.

Alzheimer's Society (2013c). Younger people with dementia. http://www.alzheimers. org.uk, accessed 16 June, 2015.

Alzheimer's Society (2014a) *Dementia UK* (2nd ed.). Alzheimer's Society: London, UK.

Alzheimer's Society (2014b) Finally a diagnosis. http://forum.alzheimers.org.uk/, accessed 3 June, 2015.

Alzheimer's Society (2014c). Depression and anxiety. http://forum.alzheimers.org.uk/, accessed 30 July, 2015.

Alzheimer's Society (2014d). Drug treatments for Alzheimer's disease. http://www. alzheimers.org.uk/, accessed 30 July, 2015.

Alzheimer's Society (2015a). Talking Point forum. http://forum.alzheimers.org.uk/, accessed 23 June, 2015.

Alzheimer's Society (2015b). Talking therapies. http://www.alzheimers.org.uk, accessed 18 August, 2015.

Alzheimer's Society (2015c). Assistive technology. http://www.alzheimers.org.uk, accessed 18 August, 2015.

Aminzadeh, F., Byszewski, A., Molnar, F. and Eisner, M. (2007). Emotional impact of dementia diagnosis: Exploring persons with dementia and caregivers' perspectives. *Aging & Mental Health*. 11(3), 281–290.

Ballard, C. and Howard, R. (2006). Neuroleptic drugs in dementia: Benefits and harm. *Nature Reviews Neuroscience*. 7, 492–500.

Ballard, C., Lana, M., Theodoulou, M., Douglas, S., McShane, R., Jacoby, R., Kossakowski, K., Yu, L. and Juszczak, E. (2008). A randomised, blinded, placebo-controlled trial in dementia patients continuing or stopping neuroleptics (The DART-AD Trial). *Nature Clinical Practice: Neurology.* 4(10), 528–529.

Ballard, C., Mohan, R., Patel, A. and Graham, C. (1994). Anxiety disorder in dementia. *Irish Journal of Psychological Medicine.* 11(3), 108–109.

Bamford, C., Lamont, S., Eccles, M., Robinson, L., May, C. and Bond, J. (2004). Disclosing a diagnosis of dementia: A systematic review. *International Journal of Geriatric Psychiatry.* 19(2), 151–169.

Barnes, T., Banerjee, S., Collins, N., Treloar, A., McIntyre, S. and Paton, C. (2012). Antipsychotics in dementia: Prevalence and quality of antipsychotic drug prescribing in UK mental health services. *British Journal of Psychiatry.* 201(3), 221–226.

Basting, A. (2006). Arts in dementia care: 'This is not the end… it's the end of this chapter'. *Generations.* 30(1), 16–20.

Beeston, D. (2006). *Older People and Suicide.* Centre for Aging and Mental Health: Stoke on Trent, England.

Bender, M. and Cheston, R. (1997). Inhabitants of a lost kingdom: A model of the subjective experiences of dementia. *Ageing & Society.* 17(5), 513–532.

Blumenthal, V. (2014). The horror of steps and stairs. http://wisewordslostforwords.wordpress.com/, accessed 22 September, 2015.

Bond, J., Stave, C., Sganga, A., Vincenzino, O., O'Connell, B. and Stanley, R.L. (2005). Inequalities in dementia care across Europe: Key findings of the Facing Dementia Survey. *International Journal of Clinical Practice.* 59, 8–14.

Bonder, B. (1994). Psychotherapy for individuals with Alzheimer disease. *Alzheimer Disease & Associated Disorders.* 8, 75–81.

Brittain, K., Corner, L., Robinson, L. and Bond, J. (2010). Ageing in place and technologies of place: The lived experience of people with dementia in changing social, physical and technological environments. *Sociology of Health and Illness.* 32(2), 272–287.

Bryden, C. (2002). A person-centred approach to counselling, psychotherapy and rehabilitation of people diagnosed with dementia in the early stages. *Dementia.* 1(2), 141–156.

Bryden, C. (2005). *Dancing with Dementia.* Jessica Kingsley Publishers: London, UK.

Camden, C. (2009). Can Gerry Robinson fix dementia care homes? Open University/BBC TV documentary.

Cheston, R., Jones, K. and Gilliard, J. (2003). Group psychotherapy and people with dementia. *Aging & Mental Health.* 7(6), 452–461.

Cheston, R. and Jones, R. (2009). A small-scale study comparing the impact of psycho-education and exploratory psychotherapy groups on newcomers to a group for people with dementia. *Aging & Mental Health.* 13(3), 420–425.

Chrisp, T.A.C., Thomas, B.D., Goddard, W.A. and Owens, A. (2011). Dementia timeline: Journeys, delays and decisions on the pathway to an early diagnosis. *Dementia.* 10(4), 555–570.

Clasper, K. (2014). Living well with Lewy Body Dementia. http://ken-kenc2.blogspot.co.uk, accessed 18 August, 2015.

Clemerson, G., Walsh, S. and Isaac, C. (2013). Towards living with young onset dementia: An exploration of coping from the perspective of those diagnosed. *Dementia: The International Journal of Social Research and Practice*. 13(4), 451–466.

Creative Dementia Arts Network. (2015). Creative minds. http://www.creativedementia.org.

Davis, R. (1989). *My Journey into Alzheimer's Disease*. Scripture Press Foundation: Harpenden, England.

Dementia Care Matters (2015). Dementia Care Matters. http://www.dementiacarematters.com/, accessed 10 August, 2015.

Dementia Friends. (2015). Dementia friends. http://blog.dementiafriends.org.uk/, accessed 17 July, 2015.

Dementia Friends (2012). Trevor Jarvis – Why I support Dementia Friends. http://blog.dementiafriends.org.uk/, accessed 22 September, 2015.

Department of Health (2009). *National Dementia Strategy*. HMSO: London, UK.

Department of Health (2012). *Prime Minister's Challenge on Dementia: Delivering Major Improvements in Dementia Care and Research by 2015*. Department of Health: London, UK.

Downs, M., Clibbens, R., Rae, C., Cook, A. and Woods, R. (2002). What do General Practitioners tell people with dementia and their families about the condition? A survey of experiences in Scotland. *Dementia*. 1, 147–158.

Duignan, D., Hedley, L. and Milverton, R. (2009). Exploring dance as a therapy for symptoms and social interaction in a dementia care unit. *Nursing Times*. 105(30), 19–22.

Ericson, A. and Eriksson, S. (2013). Intensive short-term dynamic psychotherapy in dementia: A pilot study. *International Journal of Geriatric Psychiatry*. 28(8), 877–878.

Feil, N. (2012). *The Validation Breakthrough: Simple Techniques for Communicating with People with Alzheimer's-Type Dementia* (3rd ed.). Health Professional Press: Baltimore, MD.

Friel McGowin, D. (1993). *Living in the Labyrinth*. Delacourt Press: New York.

Gainotti, G. and Marra, C. (1994). Some aspects of memory disorders clearly distinguish dementia of the Alzheimer's type from depressive pseudo-dementia. *Journal of Clinical and Experimental Neuropsychology*. 16(1), 65–78.

Glick, H. (2014). Early diagnosis fronto temporal dementia. http://earlydementiasupport.blogspot.co.uk, accessed 16 June, 2016.

Goldsmith, M. (1996). *Hearing the Voice of the Person with Dementia: Opportunities and Obstacles*. Jessica Kingsley: London, UK.

Graham, L. (2012). I'm losing my husband to a mistress called Alzheimer's. http://www.dailymail.co.uk, accessed 18 August, 2015.

Harman, G. and Clare, L. (2006). Illness representations and lived experience in early-stage dementia. *Qualitative Health Research*. 16(4), 484–502.

Hill, A. and Brettle, A. (2005). The effectiveness of counselling with older people: Results of a systematic review. *Counselling and Psychotherapy Research*. 5(4), 265–272.

Hutchinson, S.A., Leger-Krall, S. and Wilson, H.S. (1997). Early probable Alzheimer's disease and awareness context theory. *Social Science & Medicine*. 45(9), 1399–1409.

Insel, K. and Badger, T. (2002). Deciphering the 4 D's: Cognitive decline, delirium, depression and dementia – A review. *Journal of Advanced Nursing.* 38(4), 360–368.

Jones, G. (1977). A review of Feil's validation method for communicating with and caring for dementia sufferers. *Current Opinion in Psychiatry.* 10(4), 326–332.

Junaid, O. and Hegde, S. (2007). Supportive psychotherapy in dementia. *Advances in Psychiatric Treatment.* 13(1), 17–23.

Keady, J. and Nolan, M. (1995). Assessing coping responses in the early stages of dementia. *British Journal of Nursing.* 4(6), 309–314.

Kitwood, T. (1997). *Dementia Reconsidered.* Open University Press: Berkshire, England.

Kitwood, T. and Bredin, K. (1992). Towards a theory of dementia care: Personhood and well-being. *Ageing & Society.* 12, 269–287.

Leah (2007). Dementia makes concentration and comprehension tasks difficult. http://www.healthcentral.com, accessed 9 March, 2015.

McCormick, M. (2015). Truthful loving kindness. http://truthfulkindness.com/, accessed 20 June, 2015.

Mills, M. (1997). Narrative identity and dementia: A study of emotion and narrative in older people with dementia. *Ageing & Society.* 17(6), 673–698.

Mintzer, J. and Brawman-Mintzer, O. (1996). Agitation as possible expression of generalised anxiety disorder in demented elderly patients: Towards a treatment approach. *Journal of Clinical Psychiatry.* 57, 55–63.

MoMA. (2015). Meet me at MOMA. http://www.moma.org/meetme, accessed 18 August, 2015.

Neal, M. and Barton Wright, P. (2009). Validation therapy for dementia. *Cochrane Database of Systematic Reviews.* 3, CD001394.

NHS Choices (2014). Dementia: Singing for the brain. http://www.nhs.uk, accessed 15 April, 2015.

NHS Choices (2015). Getting a dementia diagnosis. http://www.nhs.uk/, accessed 15 April, 2015.

NICE (2011). Donepezil, galantamine, rivastigmine and memantine for the treatment of Alzheimer's disease. https://www.nice.org.uk, accessed 17 May, 2015.

Nichols, L. and Martindale-Adams, J. (2006). The decisive moment: Caregivers' recognition of dementia. *Clinical Gerontologist.* 30(1), 39–52.

Open University (2015). Rene Descartes – "I think, therefore I am". http://www.open.edu, accessed 23 August, 2015.

Pankhurst, B. (2014). Faces of dementia. http://www.facesofdementia.co.uk, accessed 2 March, 2015.

Phelps, R. (2014). While I still can. http://phelps2645.blogspot.co.uk, accessed 15 April, 2015.

Phinney, A. (2002). Living with the symptoms of Alzheimer's disease. In P.B. Harris (Ed.), *The Person with Alzheimer's Disease* (pp. 49–74). The Johns Hopkins University Press: Baltimore, MD.

Pinner, G. (2000). Truth-telling and the diagnosis of dementia. *British Journal of Psychiatry.* 176, 514–515.

Pratchett, T. (2008). Terry Pratchett: I'm slipping away a bit at a time... and all I can do is watch it happen. http://www.dailymail.co.uk, accessed 22 September, 2015.

Roberts, C. (2014a). My carer? My driver, my partner, my child. http://mason4233.word-press.com, accessed 16 June, 2016.

Roberts, C. (2014b). Dementia survivor, so far. https://mason4233.wordpress.com.

Rose, L. (1996). *Show Me the Way to Go Home*. Elder Books: Forest Knolls, CA.

Rusted, J., Sheppard, L. and Waller, D. (2006). A multi-centre randomized control group trial on the use of art therapy for older people with dementia. *Group Analysis*. 39, 517–536.

Sabat, S.R. (2001). *The Experience of Alzheimer's Disease*. Blackwell Publishers: Oxford, UK.

Schofield, I. and Tolson, D. (2010). *Scottish Football Museum Reminiscence Pilot Project for People with Dementia: A Realistic Evaluation*. School of Health Glasgow Caledonian University: Glasgow, Scotland.

Schweitzer, P. and Bruce, E. (2008). *Remembering Yesterday Caring Today – Reminiscence in Dementia Care: A Guide to Good Practice*. Jessica Kingsley: London, UK.

Seyfried, L., Kales, H.C., Ignacio, R.V., Conwell, Y. and Valenstein, M. (2011). Predictors of suicide in patients with dementia. *Alzheimer's and Dementia*. 7(6), 567–573.

Shankar, K. and Orrell, M. (2000). Detecting and managing depression and anxiety in people with dementia. *Current Opinion in Psychiatry*. 13(1), 55–59.

Silverfox (2014a). How does it feel to have dementia. http://parkblog-silverfox.blogspot.co.uk/, accessed 30 July, 2015.

Silverfox (2014b). Speech difficulties. http://parkblog-silverfox.blogspot.co.uk/, accessed 30 July, 2015.

Silverfox (2015a). I am worse than I seem. http://parkblog-silverfox.blogspot.co.uk/, accessed 30 July, 2015.

Silverfox (2015b). Namexa XR, take two! http://parkblog-silverfox.blogspot.co.uk/, accessed 30 July, 2015.

Speechly, C., Bridges-Webb, C. and Passmore, E. (2008). The pathway of dementia diagnosis. *Medical Journal Australia*. 189(9), 487–489.

Starkstein, S. (May 2014). Depression and suicide in dementia. Paper presented at *RANZCP Annual Congress*, Perth, Western Australia, Australia.

Swaffer, K. (2012). Prescribed disengagement. http://kateswaffer.com/, accessed 2 October, 2015.

Swaffer, K. (2013). Reactions to dementia. http://kateswaffer.com, accessed 2 October, 2015.

Swaffer, K. (2015a). Sex and dementia. http://kateswaffer.com, accessed 2 October, 2015.

Swaffer, K. (2015b). What's in a label. http://kateswaffer.com, accessed 2 October, 2015.

Swaffer, K. (2015c). Living well, living better, or living beyond dementia. https://livingbeyonddementia.wordpress.com, accessed 2 October, 2015.

Tambini, R. (2008). *A Qualitative Investigation on the Phenomenological Experience of Alzheimer's Disease from the Patient Perspective*. Massachusetts School of Professional Psychology: Newton, MA.

Taylor, R. (2007). *Alzheimer's from the Inside Out*. Health Professions Press: Baltimore, MD.

Tractenberg, R.E., Weiner, M.F., Patterson, M.B., Teri, L. and Thal, L. (2003). Comorbidity of psychopathological domains in community-dwelling persons with Alzheimer's disease. *Journal of Geriatric Psychiatry and Neurology.* 16(2), 94–99.

Vernooij-Dassen, M., Derksen, E., Scheltens, P. and Moniz-Cook, E. (2006). Receiving a diagnosis of dementia the experience over time. *Dementia.* 5(3), 397–410.

Wang, J. (2007). Group reminiscence therapy for cognitive and affective function of demented elderly in Taiwan. *International Journal of Geriatric Psychiatry.* 22(12), 1235–1240.

Watkins, R., Cheston, R., Jones, K. and Gilliard, J. (2006). 'Coming out' with Alzheimer's disease: Changes in awareness during a psychotherapy group for people with dementia. *Aging & Mental Health.* 10(2), 66–176.

Which Me Am I Today (2015). New technology – Enabling strategies for the future. https://whichmeamitoday.wordpress.com, accessed 22 September, 2015.

WHO (2015). Dementia. http://www.who.int/features/factfiles/dementia/en/, accessed 30 July, 2015.

Woods, P., Moniz-Cook, E., Lliffe, S., Campion, P., Vernooij-Dassen, M., Zanetti, O. and Franco, M. (2003). Dementia: Issues in early recognition and intervention in primary care. *Journal of the Royal Society of Medicine.* 96, 320–324.

Yalom, I. (2005). *The Theory and Practice of Group Psychotherapy* (5th ed.). Basic Books: New York.

YouTube. Gladys Wilson and Naomi Feil. https://www.youtube.com/watch?v= CrZXz10FcVM, accessed 16 June, 2016.

Zeisl, J. (2009). *I'm Still Here.* Penguin: London, UK.

PART 3

EMBRACING LIVED EXPERIENCE NARRATIVES

Narrative resources

This section includes a list of media resources where first-person narratives can be accessed. They are grouped into categories relating to the five main chapters (Chapters 3 through 7) of this book:

- Anxiety
- Depression
- Bipolar
- Psychosis
- Dementia

There is a further section covering more generic resources. These incorporate the aforementioned areas as well as other mental health issues. Please note the resources mentioned here are predominantly geared towards the United Kingdom with English-speaking examples although a wider international flavour is provided with some of the films and Internet sites. Please note full details of the films listed can be obtained from the IMDb site (http://www.imdb.com).

ANXIETY

DISCUSSION FORUMS

Anxiety Central – http://www.anxiety-central.com

Anxiety Forum – http://anxietyforum.net/forum/forum.php

Anxiety Zone – http://www.anxietyzone.com

No More Panic – http://www.nomorepanic.co.uk/forum.php

OCD Action – http://www.ocdaction.org.uk/forum

OCD UK – http://www.ocduk.org/support-forums

PTSD – https://www.myptsd.com/c

SAI (Social Anxiety Institute) – http://forum.socialanxietyinstitute.org

SAS (Social Anxiety Support) – http://www.socialanxietysupport.com/forum

SAUK (Social Anxiety UK) – http://www.social-anxiety-community.org/db

BLOGS/PERSONAL STORIES

ADAA (Anxiety and Depression Association of America) – http://www.adaa.org

Anxiety No More – http://anxietynomore.co.uk/blog

Change You Choose (PTSD) – http://changeyouchoose.com/trauma-blog

Ellen's OCD Blog – https://ellensocdblog.wordpress.com

I am Living with Anxiety – http://iamlivingwithanxiety.blogspot.co.uk

No Panic – http://www.nopanic.org.uk/category/stories

OCD UK – http://www.ocduk.org/your-ocd

Overcoming Social Anxiety – http://overcomingsocialanxiety.com/blog

Phobia Fear Release – http://www.phobia-fear-release.com/

The Beat OCD Blog – http://beatocd.blogspot.co.uk

BOOKS

Adam, D. (2015). *The Man Who Couldn't Stop: The Truth About OCD*. Picador: New York.

Breslin, N. (2015). *Me and My Mate Jeffrey: A Story of Big Dreams, Tough Realities and Facing My Demons Head On*. Hachette Books: Dublin, Ireland.

Cunningham, T. (2008). *The Hell of Social Phobia: One Man's 40 Year Struggle*. Stagedoor Publishing: London, UK.

Fields, D. (2002). Living with obsessive compulsive disorder. In R. Ramsay, A. Page, T. Godman and D. Hart (Eds.), *Changing Minds* (pp. 47–50). Gaskell: London, UK.

Ford, E., Liebowitz, M.R. and Wasmer Andrews, L. (2007). *What You Must Think of Me: A Firsthand Account of One Teenager's Experience with Social Anxiety Disorder (Adolescent Mental Health Initiative)*. Oxford University Press: Oxford, UK.

Kant, J. (2008). *The Thought that Counts: A Firsthand Account of One Teenager's Experience with Obsessive–Compulsive Disorder*. Oxford University Press: Oxford, UK.

McLean, D. (2014). *Overcoming Panic Disorder: My Story – My Journey. Into and beyond Anxiety, Panic Attacks and Agoraphobia*. Balboa: Bloomington, IN.

Smith, D. (2012). *Monkey Mind: A Memoir of Anxiety*. Simon & Shuster: New York.

Wells, J. (2006). *Touch and Go Joe*. Jessica Kingsley Publishers: London, UK.

TV

Bedlam1: Anxiety (2013) – Channel 4

Dokumenttiprojekti (2013) – BBC3

OCD Ward (2013) – ITV1

Only Human: 'Hypochondriacs: I Told You I Was Ill' (2007) – ITV1

FILMS

Adam (2009)

Amelie (2001)

As Good as It Gets (1997)

The Aviator (2004)

DEPRESSION

DISCUSSION FORUMS

Beyond Blue – https://www.beyondblue.org.au/connect-with-others/online-forums

Dealing with Depression Forum – http://www.dealingwithdepression.co.uk

Depression Chat Rooms – http://www.depression-chat-rooms.org/depression-forums.htm

Depression Fallout (For Friends and Family) – http://depressionfalloutmessageboard.yuku.com

Depression Forum – http://depressionforum.org

Mums Net (Postnatal Depression) – http://www.mumsnet.com/Talk/antenatal_postnatal_depression

BLOGS/PERSONAL STORIES

Beyond Blue – https://www.beyondblue.org.au

Daises and Bruises – http://daisiesandbruises.com

Depression Alliance – http://www.depressionalliance.org/news-blogs

Depression Blogs – http://depression-blogs-chat-rooms.org

Depression Marathon – http://depressionmarathon.blogspot.co.uk

Let's Talk about Depression – http://letstalkaboutdepression.blogspot.co.uk

Postpartum Progress – http://www.postpartumprogress.com

Storied Mind – http://www.storiedmind.com/blog

Tuxedage's Musings – https://tuxedage.wordpress.com

BOOKS

Aiken, C. (2000). *Surviving Post Natal Depression.* Jessica Kingsley Publishers: London, UK.

Brampton, S. (2008). *Shoot the Damn Dog.* Bloomsbury Publishing PLC: London, UK.

Gilman, C.P. (1892). *The Yellow Wallpaper.* Dover Publications: New York.

Haig, M. (2015). *Reasons to Stay Alive.* Canongate Books: London, UK.

Johnstone, M. (2005). *I Had a Black Dog: His Name was Depression.* Constable & Robinson Ltd.: London, UK.

Karp, D. (1996). *Speaking of Sadness: Depression, Disconnection and the Meaning of Illness.* Oxford University Press: Oxford, UK.

Kelly, R. (2014). *Black Rainbow: How Words Healed Me – My Journey through Depression.* Hodder & Stoughton: London, UK.

Lewis, G. (2006). *Sunbathing in the Rain: A Cheerful Book about Depression.* Harper Collins Publishers: London, UK.

Lott, T. (1996). *The Scent of Dried Roses*. Viking: London, UK.

Plath, S. (1963). *The Bell Jar*. Faber & Faber: London, UK.

Rice-Oxley, M. (2012). *Underneath the Lemon Tree: A Memoir of Depression and Recovery*. Little Brown: London, UK.

Serani, D. (2011). *Living with Depression: A Why Biology and Biography Matter along the Path to Hope and Healing*. Rowman & Littlefield Publishers: Plymouth, England.

Solomon, A. (2002). *The Noonday Demon: An Anatomy of Depression*. Vintage: London, UK.

Styron, W. (1990). *Darkness Visible: A Memoir of Madness*. Vintage: London, UK.

Trescothick, M. (2008). *Coming Back to Me*. Harper Collins: London, UK.

Welch, D. (2010). *Pulling Myself Together*. Sidgwick & Jackson: London, UK.

Wurtzel, E. (1994). *Prozac Nation*. Quartet Books: London, UK.

TV

Football's Suicide Secret (2013) – BBC3

Freddie Flintoff: Hidden Side of Sport (2012) – BBC1

Kerry Katona: My Depression Diaries (2013) – Channel 5

Mindgames: Depression in Sport (2009) – BBC1

Ruby Wax's Mad Confessions (2012) – Channel 4

Stacey Solomon: Depression, Teen Mums & Me (2013) – BBC3

Tonight: The Trouble with Men (2012) – ITV1

FILM

Helen (2009)

The Hours (2002)

Revolutionary Road (2008)

Sylvia (2003)

BIPOLAR

DISCUSSION FORUMS

Bipolar Support – http://www.bipolarsupport.org

Bipolar UK – http://www.bipolaruk.org.uk/e-community/DBSA

Bipolar World – http://www.bipolarworld.net/Community/bpchat.html

BP Hope – http://www.bphope.com/community

MD Junction – http://www.mdjunction.com/bipolar

Blogs/personal stories

Beautifully Broken – http://bockymama.blogspot.co.uk

Bipolar Blogging – https://bipolarblogging.wordpress.com/

Bipolar Burble – http://natashatracy.com

Bipolar: Crazy Mermaid's Blog – https://crazymer1.wordpress.com

BP Hope – http://www.bphope.com/blog

DBSA (Depression and Bipolar Support Alliance) – http://www.dbsalliance.org/site/PageServer?pagename=urgent_personal_stories

The Bipolar Griot – http://www.healthyplace.com/blogs/bipolargriot

The Secret Life of a Manic Depressive – https://thesecretlifeofamanicdepressive.word.press.com

Books

Adams, B. (2003). *The Pits and the Pendulum.* Jessica Kingsley Publishers: London, UK.

Cheney, T. (2008). *Manic.* Harper Element: London, UK.

Forney, E. (2012). *Marbles: Mania, Depression, Michelangelo and Me* (*A Graphic Memoir*). Robinson: London, UK.

Fry, S. (1997). *Moab Is My Washpot.* Arrow Books: London, UK.

Hornbacher, M. (2008). *Madness a Bipolar Life.* Harper Perennial: London, UK.

Jamison, K.R. (1995). *An Unquiet Mind.* Alfred A Knopf: New York.

Johnston, S. (2002). *The Naked Bird Watcher* (2nd ed.). The Cairn: Helensburgh, Scotland.

Pegler, J. (2004). *A Can of Madness.* Chipmunkapublishing: Brentwood, England.

Walton, N. (2013). *Bipolar Expedition.* Chipmunkapublishing: Brentwood, England.

TV

Stephen Fry: The Secret Life of the Manic Depressive (2006) – BBC2

The Madness of Prince Charming [Adam Ant] (2004) – Channel 4

Film

Bipolarized (2013)

Mr Jones (1993)

Silver Linings Playbook (2012)

The Devil and Daniel Johnstone (2005)

The Flying Scotsman (2006)

Touched with Fire (2015)

PSYCHOSIS

DISCUSSION FORUM

Hearing Voices Network – http://hvn.forumatic.com

Inter Voice – http://www.intervoiceonline.org

International Hearing Voices Network – http://www.intervoiceonline.org

Schizophrenia – http://forum.schizophrenia.com

BLOGS/PERSONAL STORIES

Female Twenty Something GSOH – http://schizophreniasucks.blogspot.co.uk

Jacqui Dillon – http://www.jacquidillon.org/blog

Living with Schizophrenia Films – http://schizophrenia24x7.com/patient-carer-video-gallery

Psychotic Depression – http://psychoticdepressionofastudent.blogspot.co.uk

BOOKS

Adamson, L. (2013). *The Voice Within: My Life with Schizophrenia*. Grosvenor House Publishing Limited: Guildford, England.

Cockburn, P. and Cockburn, H. (2011). *Henry's Demons: Living with Schizophrenia, a Father and Son Story*. Scribner: New York.

Filer, N. (2013). *The Shock of the Fall*. Harper Collins: London, UK.

Green, H. (1964). *I Never Promised You a Rose Garden*. Penguin Books: London, UK.

Hill, P. (1994). *Femme Fatale: A Personal Experience of Schizophrenia*. Autobiographical Publications: Birmingham, England.

Lamb, W. (1998). *I Know This Much is True*. Harper Collins: New York.

Romme, M., Escher, S., Dillon, J., Corstens, D. and Morris, M. (2009). *Living with Voices*. PCCS Books: Ross-on-Wye, England.

Saks, E. (2007). *The Centre Cannot Hold – A Memoir of My Schizophrenia*. Virago: London, UK.

Schiller, L. (1994). *The Quiet Room*. Warner Books: New York.

Steele, K. (2002). *The Day the Voices Stopped*. Basic Books: New York.

TV

Bedlam 3: Psychosis (2013) – Channel 4

My Name Is Alan and I Paint Pictures (2007) – Sky Arts 1

Tulisa: My Mum and Me (2010) – BBC3

FILM

A Beautiful Mind (2001)

Das Weisse Rauschen (*The White Sound*) (2001)

K-Pax (2001)

Lek Wysokosci (*Fear of Falling*) (2011)

Shine (1996)

Some Voices (2000)

The Soloist (2009)

Through a Glass Darkly (1961)

DEMENTIA

DISCUSSION FORUMS

Aging Care – https://www.agingcare.com/Alzheimers-Dementia/Discussions-1

Alz Connected – https://www.alzconnected.org

Alzheimer's Society Talking Point – http://forum.alzheimers.org.uk/forum.php

Lewy Body Dementia Association – http://www.lbda.org/phpbbforum

FTD Support Forum – http://www.ftdsupportforum.com

BLOGS/PERSONAL STORIES

Creating Life with Words – http://kateswaffer.com/2013/03/29/reactions-to-dementia

Dementia Survivor So Far – https://mason4233.wordpress.com

Faces of Dementia – http://www.facesofdementia.co.uk

FTD (Fronto Temporal Dementia) Dementia Support blog – http://earlydementiasupport.blogspot.co.uk

Living Well with Lewy Body Disease – http://ken-kenc2.blogspot.co.uk

Living with Passion (A Huntingdon's Disease Journey) – http://livingwithpassion90.blogspot.co.uk/2015_03_01_archive.html

Truthful Loving Kindness – http://truthfulkindness.com

Sharing My Life with Lewy Body Dementia – http://parkblog-silverfox.blogspot.co.uk

Which Me Am I Today – https://whichmeamitoday.wordpress.com/blog

While I Still Can – http://phelps2645.blogspot.co.uk

Wise Words Lost Forever – https://wisewordslostforwords.wordpress.com

Young Dementia UK – http://www.youngdementiauk.org/resources/blogs

BOOKS

Bernlef, J. (1988). *Out of Mind*. Faber & Faber: London, UK.

Bryden, C. (2005). *Dancing with Dementia*. Jessica Kingsley Publishers: London, UK.

Davis, R. (1989). *My Journey into Alzheimer's Disease*. Scripture Press Foundation: Harpenden, England.

Friel McGowin, D. (1993). *Living in the Labyrinth*. Delacourt Press: New York.

Rose, L. (1996). *Show Me the Way to Go Home*. Elder Books: Forest Knolls, CA.

Sabat, S.R. (2001). *The Experience of Alzheimer's Disease*. Blackwell Publishers: Oxford, UK.

Stokes, G. (2010). *And Still the Music Plays: Stories of People with Dementia* (2nd ed.). Hawker Publication: London, UK.

Taylor, R. (2007). *Alzheimer's from the Inside Out*. Health Professions Press: Baltimore, MD.

TV

Can Gerry Robinson Fix Dementia Care Homes (2009) – BBC2

Louis Theroux: Extreme Love – Dementia (2012) – BBC1

Malcolm and Barbara: Love's Farewell (2007) – ITV1

Mum, Dad, Alzheimer's and Me (2009) – Channel 4

My Life on a Post It Note (2006) – BBC1

Terry Pratchett Living with Alzheimer's (2009) – BBC2

Tonight: Living with Dementia (2014) – ITV1

Wonderland: The Alzheimer's Choir (2009) – BBC2

FILM

Aurora Borealis (2006)

Away from Her (2006)

En Sång för Martin (*A Song for Martin*) (2001)

Firefly Dreams (2001)

Iris (2001)

Maine Gandhi Ko Nahin Mara (*I Did Not Kill Gandhi*) (2005)

Still Alice (2015)

The Notebook (2004)

The Savages (2007)

U Me Aur Hum [*You, Me and Us*] (2008)

GENERIC

Discussion forums

Blueboard – https://blueboard.anu.edu.au

Healing Well – http://www.healingwell.com/community

Health Boards – http://www.healthboards.com/boards

Mental Health Forum – http://www.mentalhealthforum.net/forum

Patient – http://patient.info/forums

Sane – http://sane.org.uk/support_forum/index.php

Sober Recovery – http://www.soberrecovery.com/forums

Young Minds – http://www.youngminds.org.uk

Blogs/personal stories

Curiously Creative (*Digital Stories*) – http://curiositycreative.org.uk

Headspace – https://www.headspace.com/blog/category/5/user-stories

Health Central – http://www.healthcentral.com

Healthtalk – http://www.healthtalk.org

Healthy Place – http://www.healthyplace.com/alzheimers

Mind (*Your Stories*) – http://www.mind.org.uk/information-support/your-stories

My Invisible Life – http://www.myinvisiblelife.net/our-storytellers

The Site – http://www.thesite.org/your-stories

Time to Change – http://www.time-to-change.org.uk/join-the-conversation

Turn to Me – https://turn2me.org/group-support

Young Minds – http://www.youngminds.org.uk/for_children_young_people/real_stories

Your Stories – http://www.leedsandyorkpft.nhs.uk/about_us/publications/your_stories

Books

Camus, A. (1982). *The Outsider*. Penguin: London, UK.

Eugenides, J. (2012). *The Marriage Plot*. Fourth Estate: London, UK.

Grant, S. (1996). *The Passion of Alice*. Sceptre: London, UK.

Grass, G. (1993). *The Tin Drum*. Vintage: London, UK.

Hesse, H. (1955). *Steppenwolf*. Penguin: London, UK.

Lamb, W. (1992). *She's Come Undone*. Simon & Shuster: London, UK.

Salinger, J.D. (1945). *Catcher in the Rye*. Penguin: London, UK.

Sayer, P. (1988). *The Comforts of Madness*. Constable & Company Ltd: London, UK.

Woolf, V. (1925). *Mrs Dalloway*. Harper Press: London, UK.

Yates, R. (1975). *Disturbing the Peace*. Vintage: London, UK.

TV

A World of Pain: Meera Syal on Self Harm (2009) – BBC2

Bedlam 2: Crisis (2013) – Channel 4

Bedlam 4: Breakdown (2013) – Channel 4

Diaries of a Broken Mind (2013) – BBC3

Don't Call Me Crazy (2013) – BBC3

Jodie Marsh: Bullied (2012) – Channel 5

Living with Alcohol (2010) – BBC1

Louis Theroux: By Reason of Insanity (2015) – BBC1

My Big Fat Diary (2013) – Channel 4

Piers Morgan's Life Stories: Dame Kelly Holmes (2012) – ITV1

Takin' Over the Asylum (1994) – BBC2

FILM

Black Swan (2010)

Interiors (1978)

K-Pax (2001)

Life Is Sweet (1990)

The Man with Golden Arm (1955)

Thin (2006)

Trainspotting (1996)

What's Eating Gilbert Grape (1993)

ADDITIONAL RESOURCES

ARTS FESTIVALS

Little Sparks – http://littlesparks.rocks

Livewell Arts Festival – http://www.plymouthcommunityhealthcare.co.uk/livewell/livewell-home-page/livewell-arts-festival1

Love Arts – http://loveartsleeds.co.uk

NI Mental Health Arts and Film Festival – http://www.nimhaff.org

Scottish Mental Health Arts and Film Festival – http://www.mhfestival.com

HELP AND ADVICE

Age Exchange – http://www.age-exchange.org.uk

Alzheimer's Association – http://www.alz.org/

Alzheimer's Society – http://www.alzheimers.org.uk

B-eat – http://www.b-eat.co.uk

Bipolar UK – http://www.bipolaruk.org.uk

CALM – *http://www.thecalmzone.net/*

Choices in Recovery – http://www.choicesinrecovery.com

Cruse Bereavement care – http://www.cruse.org.uk

Dementia Friends – https://www.dementiafriends.org.uk

Drink Aware – http://www.drinkaware.co.uk

Maytree (*A Sanctuary for the Suicidal*) – http://www.maytree.org.uk

Mental Health Foundation – http://www.mentalhealth.org.uk

Mind – http://www.mind.org.uk

National Self Harm network – http://www.nshn.co.uk

NHS Choices – http://www.nhs.uk/Pages/HomePage.aspx

Papyrus (*Prevention of Young Suicide*) – https://www.papyrus-uk.org

Rape Crisis – http://www.rapecrisis.org.uk

Rethink Mental Illness – http://www.rethink.org

Samaritans – http://www.samaritans.org

Sane – http://www.sane.org.uk

Self Harm – http://www.selfharm.org.uk

Support Line – http://www.supportline.org.uk/problems/index.php

Survivors of Suicide – http://www.survivorsofsuicide.com/index.html

The Bereavement Trust – http://bereavement-trust.org.uk

Time to Change – http://www.time-to-change.org.uk

Learning strategy

This chapter provides readers with a framework for accessing and processing media narratives which convey lived mental health experience. The strategy for learning outlined addresses a continuous, cyclical process of learning with specific points of engagement – before, during and after the accessing of media narratives as shown in Figure 9.1 (Morris, 2015). It is aimed at teaching personnel, workplace trainers and healthcare learners providing a structure developed around Kolb's (1984) experiential cycle with learning and reflection progressively refined through successive events. Various learning theories are highlighted relating to processes and dynamics operating throughout this learning cycle.

SECTION 1: STRATEGY FOR LEARNING

BEFORE

This stage is concerned with the careful selection of narratives and the preparation of learners for accessing the content carried.

PREPARATION OF LEARNERS

Introduce related theoretical concepts connected with narrative themes

When accessing lived experience narratives and embracing their learning potential, there is a need to be mindful of individuals' previous and current learning. This reflects Ausubel's (2000) assimilation theory which sees new material being anchored to a base of already established learning. From a mental health perspective it might be timely, for example, to help learners understand what schizophrenia is before viewing films such as *Some Voices* or *A Beautiful Mind*. This might initially be geared towards dispelling myths about this condition and understanding diagnostic criteria, epidemiology and treatment approaches.

Establish preferences regarding learning styles and media source types

The importance here is in acknowledging how students learn with consideration shown to individual preferences and needs (Honey and Mumford, 1982; Kolb, 1984). Flemming's (2001) visual, auditory, reading and kinaesthetic (VARK) framework can also be applied reviewing how certain media source types resonate more with different people. It can also be noted that the depth and range of learning can be influenced by the type of media product selected. This was shown in Morris's (2014) study which found audiovisual resources being the most memorable and impactful whilst autobiographical narratives

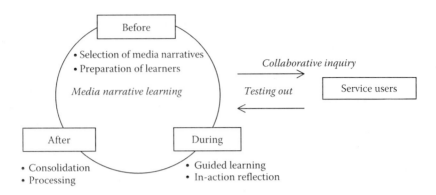

Figure 9.1 Learning strategy. (From Morris, G., Creating a strategy of learning: Engaging with mental health lived experience through the use of media narratives, PhD thesis, University of Huddersfield, Huddersfield, England, 2015.)

carried greater depth of expressiveness. Whilst the Internet provided a wealth of information, there was a tendency for participants to feel overwhelmed highlighting the need for structured guidance.

Outline relevance of narratives to be accessed to current learning

The preparation here concerns alerting learners to what it is they will be accessing and which aspects in particular to attend to. The Gestalt theory principle of *figure and ground* shows how certain elements can be 'drawn out' and attended to relegating other parts to the background (Köhler, 1947). This is also the 'selling' point, providing learners with a rationale or need for the material about to be accessed.

SELECTION OF NARRATIVES

The number of accessible narratives is vast, and it is only possible to sample a very small fraction of the total range. Consideration should also be shown to the potential of learners feeling overwhelmed or saturated by personal accounts of distress. Attention is therefore needed with regards to the number and type of products selected, the frequency with which they are accessed and opportunities for processing narratives and gaining support. The selection of lived experience narratives can be made according to certain criteria:

Experience type

Range – Collectively acknowledges the uniqueness of each person's lived experience.
Balance – Examples selected from across the lived experience spectrum of
  struggling-coping.
Representativeness – Narratives can be related to others' mental health experience.
Seldom encountered – Provides important opportunities for learning around mental
  health issues infrequently encountered through practice.
Stigmatising – These can be examined along with health promotional examples generating discussion around core themes.

Learning

Immediacy – Can engage recipients in the *here and now*
Emotional impact – Memorable and attention 'grabbing'
Core learning themes – Provide significant themes for review
Cultural and contextual issues – Reflect the perspective/dynamic within which different
    people experience their lives

Accessibility

This section concerns the physical accessibility of media narratives as well as recipients'
ability to make sense of relayed messages.

Freely accessible – Narrative products can be easily obtained for learning purposes.
Narrative – Concerns the articulateness and expressive ability of narrators.
Differing channels of communication – Includes audiovisual, textual and interactive
    examples from the full scope of media types.
Creative modes – Visual messages, auditory cues and symbolism conveyed, especially
    with regards to a person's communicative impairment.

DURING

This part involves a guided learning process, supervising and supporting learners with
their processing of personal narratives. It is concerned with helping learners identify and
attend to core learning themes present in what is being expressed. This can be reflected
through Gestalt theory and the concept of making sense of the *unified whole* (Köhler,
1947). Broadbent's (1958) filter theory can also be applied showing how selective individuals' attention can be and the need to accentuate core learning themes. It is also vital to
ensure that learners are sufficiently supported throughout this process with a containing
environment offered on account of the potential for feeling distressed or overwhelmed.
As shown by the work of Pavlov (2003), positive or negative associations can be formed
during the learning process which includes the climate of learning. High levels of distress
or unease with regards to people's narratives can cause learners to psychologically withdraw for self-protection.

NARRATIVE ACTIVITY

Guided processing – Aiding the learning process through highlighting core themes to
    attend to. This is assisted by associated resources (i.e. worksheets, guided study
    material and questions).
Reflection in action – Discussion and processing of themes during the activity. This stim-
    ulates the ability to process experience whilst engaged in the present (Schön, 1983).
Sensitivity and support – Able to respond to potential emotional distress experienced by
    students.

PROCESS ISSUES

Timing – Consideration needs to be shown for the timing and frequency of when narra-
    tives are offered.

Overload potential – Relates to both content and emotional aspects.

Supportive learning environment – Creation of an environment conducive to learning (Maslow, 1970).

Immediacy – Offered through *here and now* examples.

Modelled engagement – Ways of engaging with narrative material demonstrated (Bandura, 1977).

AFTER

This part follows the accessing of media narratives and is concerned with processing learning and supporting students. It provides opportunities to revisit previously introduced learning themes and progressively refine understanding as illustrated through Argyris and Schön's (1978) double loop learning process.

PROCESSING

Reflection on action – Discussion and processing of themes *after* the activity (Schön, 1983)

Highlight core learning themes – Reiteration and summary of key learning material

Reframing – Opportunities to look at alternative reading of people's behaviour based upon understanding of lived experience

Reprocessing – Re-examination of previously introduced theoretical material

Introduction of new theoretical material – Further development and progression of learning

PROCESS APPROACH

Modelled approach – Learners provided with a 'guide' to processing narratives (Bandura, 1977)

Sensitivity – Shown to personal experience shared in narratives

Saturation – Awareness of potential information/emotion overload

Supportive engagement – Provided for learners in terms of generated emotions

Reflective approach – Promotion of critical, questioning ability

'TESTING OUT'

As the diagram in Figure 9.2 illustrates, the focus upon media lived experience narratives is only part of learners' overall accessing of personal stories. It is complemented through the inclusion of service users within classroom learning (see Chapter 2) and opportunities gained through practice contact. The essence concerns the ability by learners and practitioners to 'test out' their developing understanding which is most effectively done *with* and not *on* service users.

SERVICE USER COLLABORATION

Facilitate opportunities – For service user involvement in student learning

Promote opportunities – For learner engagement with service users

Model 'testing out' – Demonstrating collaborative development of understanding *with* service users (Bandura, 1977)

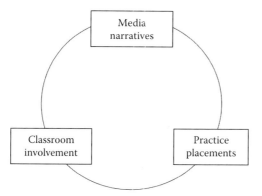

Figure 9.2 Service user narratives – *the unified whole.*

Practice reflection – Opportunities for sharing and discussing practice encounters
Consolidation – Further processing of learning with service users through appropriate
    channels, that is, designated discussion forums

PROCESS APPROACH

Agency involvement – Promotion and development of higher levels of service user
    engagement within educational settings (Tew et al., 2004)
Service user support – Support provided regarding the emotional impact of narrative
    sharing. Negotiation of communicative approaches available for sharing 'stories'
Student support – Promoting approaches for working *with* service users and facilitating
    narrative expression

WIDER COLLABORATION AND ENGAGEMENT

Multi-agency collaboration – Fostering opportunities for narrative sharing involving
    service users, educational staff, healthcare professionals and media personnel
Facilitated narrative expression – Offering creative means for those with communicative
    deficits (i.e. cognitive impairment)
Health promotion – Involvement with arts festivals, community workshops and school
    promotions
Scholarship/research – Collaboration with service users on academic and research
    projects

SECTION 2: LEARNING APPROACHES

This part outlines a range of activities and learning approaches which can be carried out
either individually or in groups concerning engagement with lived experience. They are
designed to help structure training and learning approaches which can be carried out in
either educational or clinical settings. Whilst specific narrative products are indicated
with some of the activities, they can be easily modified to include alternative examples
as desired.

FILM NARRATIVES

WATCHING *IRIS*

The chosen film *Iris* (Fox et al., 2001) features Judy Dench as the celebrated writer Iris Murdoch. It showcases the impact that dementia has upon a person to whom 'words' are highly significant. It is also concerned with the impact that her deteriorating cognition has upon her husband John Bayley and their relationship together as a couple.

Watching *Iris*: Worksheet

Before watching the film

What do I feel could be the felt/lived experience of

- People who have dementia?
- Close relatives/carers of those with dementia?

Whilst watching the film

- What sense do we get of Iris and her lived experience?
- What sense do we get of her husband John's lived experience?
- What impact does the condition dementia have upon their relationship?

After the watching the film

- To what degree have your values, beliefs and attitudes been influenced by watching this film?

CULTURAL LEARNING

International films are selected according to the cultural groups that learners are likely to encounter in practice. Within the author's geographical area of West Yorkshire, for example, this can include Afro-Caribbean, South East Asian and Eastern European cultures. The example given here concerns the Polish film *Lek Wysokosci* (*Fear of Falling*) (Bromski et al., 2011), although many other examples can be substituted. This film is about a young father to be (Tomasz) whose father (Wojciech) is diagnosed with schizophrenia. It explores the impact that this has upon each of them as well as their relationship together.

Cultural learning: Eastern European perspectives on mental health

Preparatory learning

- Introductory information given around the condition and experience of schizophrenia
- Speakers invited to talk with learners about Polish/Eastern European culture and perspectives upon mental health issues
- Learners given brief information about the film to be watched

Watching the film
Screening of film *Lek Wysokosci*

Discussion of themes
Students asked to consider
    The impact that schizophrenia has upon Tomasz and Wojciech as well as their relationship together
    Differences in attitudes and care interventions seen in the film with what learners have observed in the United Kingdom

Follow-up
Summing up of exercise with further theoretical material and narrative accounts accessed

READING THE NEWS

GAZING BEHIND THE HEADLINES

This activity is geared at getting student to think beyond the 'facts' given in news stories/ headlines and to consider what the personal perspective might be.

Gazing behind the headlines

'1200 killed by mental patients' – *The Sun* newspaper (Parry and Moyes, 2013)
    Students asked to read this story and discuss their thoughts and feelings about the headlines and content.

Exercise
Students given time to locate the following:

Research/statistics around

- Number of people killed or harmed by those *with* diagnosed mental health problems
- Number of people killed or harmed by those *without* diagnosed mental health problems
- Number of people experiencing mental health problems harmed, intimidated or victimised

Discussion and sharing
Opportunity for learners to share and process their findings

Consolidation
Review of reports, studies and personal narratives reflecting the impact that stigmatising public attitudes have upon those experiencing mental health problems

MAGAZINE FEATURES

This activity asks learners to find magazine articles relating personal mental health narratives. A range of titles from the pricier, more substantial types to the cheap 'coffee table' examples can be offered. Teen magazines can also be included. Individual/small groups are allocated specific types covering a range of what is accessible.

Magazine features

Two weeks before the activity – learners are allocated magazine types and asked to locate stories of personal mental health experience.

Group work
Opportunity given in small groups to discuss examples

One of these is selected to feed back concerning

- The related mental health experience
- Magazine title and targeted audience
- The reliability of the information narrated

Discussion
Related themes discussed with fellow students

READING BOOKS

The exercises shown here utilise examples from autobiographical and fictional narratives. The former can be found in abundance detailing wide ranging mental health experience. The latter include some intriguing examples dating back many years such as Jonathan Swift's (1704) *Tale of a tub*. In some instances the work can be regarded as semi-autobiographical. Both types of narrative indicated here can be offered to learners as full or partial texts.

REFRAMING OBSERVED BEHAVIOUR

Learners are given a selected chapter to read which highlights some of the difficulties faced by the narrator on account of his cognitive deterioration. A number of these difficulties could be regarded by others as 'problematic' or 'challenging' behaviours. Reading this narrative though allows us to *reframe* and understand these aspects from a lived and felt perspective.

Reframing observed behaviour: *My Journey into Alzheimer's Disease* (Davis, 1989)

Chapter 7 – The Abnormal Changes so far

Worksheet

- What sense do you make of the difficulties experienced by the narrator?
- How might these experiences affect his subsequent behaviour or engagement with others?

- How might his observed behaviour be perceived by others if unaware of his internal dynamics?
- Consider ways in which he could be best supported to cope with these difficulties.

Group work

- Opportunity provided for learners to share thoughts about the narrator's internal dementia experience.

Reframing exercise

- Learners asked to draw up a list of as many 'challenging behaviours' that they can think of which might be encountered within dementia care.
- Possible internal dynamics/drivers are now added to each of these behaviours.

Consolidation

- Learners introduced to O'Connor and Seymour's (1990) interpersonal model illustrating links between internal response and external behaviour.
- Further narrative examples provided.

REFRAMING LANGUAGE (EMOTIONAL CONTENT)

Reframing language (emotional content)

Learners are given selected extracts from the following texts which provide examples of disordered/distorted thinking:

I never promised you a rose garden – Hannah Green (1964).
Briefing for a descent into hell – Doris Lessing (1971).
The yellow wallpaper – Joanne Perkins Gilman (1892).

They are then asked to identify what *emotions* are being conveyed through the narrative.

Discussion/processing
Opportunities given to discuss thoughts with fellow students about validating what is conveyed on a *feelings* level.

Follow-up
Consolidation of learning through the reviewing of personal narratives from individuals reflecting upon their feelings when experiencing altered cognition.

WATCHING TV

There are many mental health narratives carried within TV programmes covering a spectrum from entertainment to education. The varied genres include documentaries, news items, drama programmes, soaps and reality TV. The two types selected here concern the documentary (educational) and soap (entertainment) format of which there are many examples broadcast on a weekly basis. They can also be accessed from various online video streaming resources, that is, BBCi player, ITV player, 4 On Demand, YouTube or Box of Broadcasts.

FLY ON THE WALL: WATCHING DOCUMENTARIES

The example chosen here is the BBC documentary *Mindgames: Depression in sport* (Hughes, 2009). It features a selection of high profile sports personalities sharing their personal experiences of depression.

Fly on the wall: Watching documentaries

Preparation

- Students given introductory information relating to the condition and experience of depression.
- Worksheet developed guiding learners through core themes to focus on *whilst* watching the programme. This covers
  - 'What do they have to be depressed about?'
  - Expectations, stress and pressure
  - The sporting culture and available opportunities for sharing

Watch documentary
The programme is paused after individual narratives to allow time to write down worksheet responses.

Group work
Learners allocated time to discuss thoughts around questions/themes identified in the worksheet.

Consolidation
Opportunity provided to feedback and discuss key issues.

Review of further range of narratives by sports personalities around feelings of depression.

WATCHING THE SOAPS

Watching the soaps: Stacey Slater/Eastenders

Preparation
Students given background information about the condition and experience of individuals with bipolar.

Introductory details provided about the character Stacey Slater.

Students given clips to watch illustrating Stacey's bipolar experience, for example, '*Stacey gets sectioned*':
https://www.youtube.com/watch?v=L6aTix8P9yQ

Watching the programme
Students enabled to watch selected clips.

Discussion/processing
Opportunities given to examine how Stacey's experience is depicted and the impact upon her and others around her. Particular emphasis is given to how different characters might be feeling.

Consolidation
Narrative extracts from others who have had related experiences are reviewed such as Neil Walton's (2013) *Bipolar Expedition*.

SURFING THE INTERNET

There are countless options here for finding personal narratives on the Internet. A key issue concerns the sifting through the plethora of available resources and avoiding becoming lost or overwhelmed. This is where clear guidance can be very beneficial. A starting place can involve searching for specific service user/mental health advocacy groups which generally feature personal narratives. Other useful locations include social media sites or resources such as YouTube. The examples featured here illustrate two rich types of resource – discussion forums and blogs.

DISCUSSION FORUMS

Discussion forums: Anxiety

Allocation of discussion forums
Discussion forums are divided amongst individual learners/small groups as related to problems with anxiety (see Chapter 8).

Allocation of themes
Selected learning themes given, for example, *receiving a diagnosis, taking medication, requesting help or supporting others*.

Searching
Learners allocated time to review postings and discussion threads relating to allocated themes.

Processing
Opportunity provided for learners to feed back findings and discuss with fellow learners.

READING BLOGS

> **Reading blogs: Dementia blogs**
>
> *Allocation of blogs*
> Selected examples given to students/small groups such as Howard Glick, Silverfox or Kate Swaffer (see Chapter 8).
> These are carefully selected according to the depth and range of information posted.
>
> *Allocate themes/questions*
> Learners to identify and summarise what are individuals saying concerning the allocated themes.
>
> *Feedback*
> Online sharing resource set up for students to post their responses/thoughts
> Time provided for learners to review work from other groups.
>
> *Group discussion*
> Opportunity given to process and discuss learning from blog narratives.

OTHER EXAMPLES

To complement the examples suggested earlier, there are many other innovative and engaging exercises which can be offered. This can involve a diverse range of media types including videogames, radio programmes, painting, sculpture, graphic novels and theatre performances. There are an increasing number of mental health arts festivals (see Chapter 8) which provide ideal opportunities for learners to access narrative experience presented through many different expressive modes. When it comes to accessing narrative examples, individuals need only be constrained by the limits of their imagination.

REFERENCES

Argyris, C. and Schön, D. (1978). *Organizational Learning: A Theory of Action Perspective.* Addison-Wesley Publishing Co.: Reading, MA.

Ausubel, D. (2000). *The Acquisition and Retention of Knowledge: A Cognitive View.* Springer Science + Business Media: London, UK.

Bandura, A. (1977). *Social Learning Theory.* Prentice Hall: Englewood Cliffs, NJ.

Broadbent, D. (1958). *Perception and Communication.* Pergamon Press: London, UK.

Bromski, J., Gajewski, D., Jastrzebska, E. and Konopka, B. (2011). *Lek Wysokosci.* Kanibal Films Distribution: Poland.

Davis, R. (1989). *My Journey into Alzheimer's Disease.* Scripture Press Foundation: Harpenden, England.

Flemming, N. (2001). *Teaching and Learning Styles: Vark Strategies.* Neil D. Flemming: Christchurch, New Zealand.

Fox, R., Rudin, S. and Eyre, R. (2001). *Iris*. BBC: London, UK.

Gilman, C.P. (1892). *The Yellow Wallpaper*. Dover Publications: New York.

Green, H. (1964). *I Never Promised You a Rose Garden*. Penguin Books: London, UK.

Honey, P. and Mumford, A. (1982). *Manual of Learning Styles*. P Honey: London, UK.

Hughes, R. (2009). *Mindgames: Depression in Sport*. BBC: London, UK.

Köhler, W. (1947). *Gestalt Psychology: The Definitive Statement of the Gestalt Theory*. Liveright Publishing Corporation: New York.

Kolb, D.A. (1984). *Experiential Learning: Experience as the Source of Learning and Development*. Prentice-Hall: Englewood Cliffs, NJ.

Lessing, D. (1971). *Briefing for a Descent into Hell*. Panther: Suffolk, England.

Maslow, A. (1970). *Motivation and Personality*. Harper: New York.

Morris, G. (2014). Developing awareness and understanding amongst mental health nursing students of the lived experience of dementia with the aid of selected first-person media resources. *Journal of Research in Nursing*. 19(5), 434–448.

Morris, G. (2015). Creating a strategy of learning: Engaging with mental health lived experience through the use of media narratives. PhD thesis. University of Huddersfield: Huddersfield, England.

O'Connor, J. and Seymour, J. (1990). *Introducing Neuro-Linguistic Programming – Psychological Skills for Understanding and Influencing People*. Aquarian: London, UK.

Parry, R. and Moyes, S. (7 October 2013). 1200 Killed by mental patients. *The Sun*. Retrieved from http://www.thesun.co.uk, accessed 15 October, 2015.

Pavlov, I.P. (2003). *Conditioned Reflexes*. Dover Publications: New York.

Schön, D. (1983). *The Reflective Practitioner. How Professionals Think in Action*. Basic Books: New York.

Swift, J. (1704). *A Tale of a Tub*. George Routledge & Sons: London, UK.

Tew, J., Gell, C. and Foster, F. (2004). *A Good Practice Guide: Learning from Experience: Involving Service Users and Carers in Mental Health Education and Training*. Mental Health in Higher Education, NIMH: Nottingham, England.

Walton, N. (2013). *Bipolar Expedition*. Chipmunkapublishing: Brentwood, England.

So what?

It has been the intention that mental health practitioners and learners reading this text become more mindful and questioning about the internal experience (thoughts and feelings) of those they are working with. This concerns the promotion of more reflective and challenging approaches to practice. Whilst the themes around *lived experience* covered in this text are based upon an extensive range of narratives, it needs reiterating that no claims are made that the totality of mental health experience has been captured or anything close to it. It might therefore be the case that some readers feel that important details have been missed or overlooked. This would no doubt still be so if this work was extended considerably or perhaps focused upon a *single* mental health issue. We can consider here the billions of people affected worldwide with mental health issues, each with their own personal narrative to relate. It can also be noted that a person's perception of experience is subject to changes, along with alterations in their mental health state. Very different accounts can be given by the same person depending upon the point in their mental health journey that stories are shared. All of these issues demonstrate the need for practitioners to put aside their expectations when working with service users and facilitate expression around internal experience. What is important is that practitioners become more thoughtful and questioning, testing out their developing insights *with* individual service users and not *on* them. It is not the intention that readers reviewing this text can claim to understand mental health experience in all its vast complexity, but more so to be inspired sufficiently by this work to continue with their journey of discovery.

Chapters 1 and 2 set the scene for this work defining concepts of *lived experience* and *narrative* as well as providing some of the contextual issues regarding service user involvement in healthcare education. Each of the main Chapters 3 through 7, focused around mental health experience, has been divided into three distinct sections. Section 1 is concerned with what it *feels like* to live with and experience mental health issues. This provides a window through which to view a person's internal world as well as gaining contextual understanding of the wider influencing factors. The nature of one's mental health experience has been addressed from a holistic perspective, with consideration shown to the dynamically different ways in which a person can be affected. This acknowledgement of internal experience facilitates a more empathic as opposed to sympathetic approach being utilised. Section 2 embraces what it feels like to be on the receiving end of interventions, creating a better understanding around the relevance or significance of care approaches to each person. This promotes awareness around areas where people are having difficulties engaging with care. People can easily be judged as 'non-compliant' and viewed unfavourably for not engaging with the help offered. If taking the time to explore a person's feelings and thoughts, we might appreciate the dilemma or difficulty they are facing. Medication side effects such as weight gain, fuzzy thinking or sexual dysfunction can be particularly distressing. Alternatively, taking medication can act as an unwelcome signifier that a person has mental health problems. Whilst these reasons can be frowned upon by some when weighed up against an intervention's potential benefits, it is through the 'hearing' of personal narratives that we become much more understanding of the dynamics involved. It has also been an intention of this work to reflect a more balanced view of mental health experience across a *struggling–coping* continuum. Criticisms can be levelled at the predominant attention upon deficits, problems and losses instead of coping skills and personal qualities. Section 3 is concerned with *well-being*, reflecting aspects such as resilience and recovery as well as showing how differently a person can regard their overall mental health experience. It is noted that a number of individuals regard their mental health experience, though at times being seriously debilitating, as an important catalyst for change. Chapter 8 illustrates the breadth of narrative source types with a selection of examples for different mental health states provided. The final chapter is concerned with the engagement with lived experience narratives as part of a learning process. A learning strategy is outlined along with a range of educational activities.

Peer support has emerged as a significant factor in a person's recovery and is in need of further study to examine the evidence. Peer support groups, blogs and discussion forums play a vital part in a person's recovery. This facilitates feelings of connection and engagement with other 'experts by experience', individuals who can relate to a person's experience. There is also a key need being met through the opportunity to support others, helping one feel purposeful, needed and valued. This was reflected by interviewees' responses (Chapter 2) around their involvement in healthcare education. There are evidently many mutual benefits through attending to service user narratives which can be both therapeutic and educational. This is recognised by a number of service user agency groups who promote opportunities for volunteers to share personal mental health experience with others. It should be noted that anyone, no matter how communicatively impaired they might seem, has a narrative worth sharing. The main thing is that we keep trying to connect with service users, working *with* them to find the most appropriate and vibrant means of telling their story. It is worth the effort because the benefits can be huge.

Index